FAST METABOLISM
FOOD RX

FAST METABOLISM
FOOD RX

7 POWERFUL PRESCRIPTIONS TO
FEED YOUR BODY BACK TO HEALTH

Haylie Pomroy

with Eve Adamson

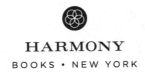

HARMONY
BOOKS • NEW YORK

HAYLIE
POMROY

The material in this book is for informational purposes only and not intended as a substitute for the advice and care of your physician. As with all new weight loss or weight maintenance regimes, the nutrition and fitness program described in this book should be followed only after first consulting with your physician to make sure it is appropriate for your individual circumstances. Keep in mind that nutritional needs vary from person to person, depending on age, sex, health status, and total diet. The author and the publisher expressly disclaim responsibility for any adverse effects that may result from the use or application of the information contained in this book.

Published in the United States by Harmony Books, an imprint of the Crown Publishing Group, a division of Penguin Random House LLC, New York.
www.crownpublishing.com

Harmony Books is a registered trademark, and the Circle colophon is a trademark of Penguin Random House LLC.

Library of Congress Cataloging-in-Publication Data
Names: Pomroy, Haylie, author. | Adamson, Eve, author.
Title: Fast metabolism food Rx : 7 powerful prescriptions to feed your body back to health / Haylie Pomroy, Eve Adamson.
Description: First edition. | New York : Harmony, [2016]
Identifiers: LCCN 2015033348 | ISBN 9780804141079 (hardcover) | ISBN 9780804141086 (eISBN)
Subjects: LCSH: Nutrition. | Diet therapy. | Food preferences. | Metabolism—Regulation. | BISAC: HEALTH & FITNESS / Diets. | HEALTH & FITNESS / Nutrition | HEALTH & FITNESS / Women's Health.
Classification: LCC RA784 .P646 2016 | DDC 613.2—dc23 LC record available at http://lccn.loc.gov/2015033348

ISBN 978-0-8041-4107-9
eBook ISBN 978-0-8041-4108-6

PRINTED IN THE UNITED STATES OF AMERICA

Jacket design by Jenny Carrow
Front jacket photography by Albuquerque/iStock

10 9 8 7 6 5 4 3 2 1

First Edition

I dedicate this book to the very first love of my life: a drug called

prednisone. If it were not for the relief you afforded me, and the

health crisis you left me in, I never would have found my true love,

which is helping others navigate their way. I also dedicate this book to

my mom, Dr. Jeanne Wilson, because when I was diagnosed,

her response was, "Don't worry about it. You're smart.

I know you will figure this out."

Contents

Introduction:
The Making of a Body
Whisperer

You never know how strong you are until being strong is the only choice you have.
   —Commonly attributed to Bob Marley

Every time you eat food, you trigger internal changes within your metabolism. Just the physical acts of eating, smelling, and tasting food activate metabolic pathways that ignite gene expression. They also signal the body to distribute sugars, stimulate hormone secretion, and regulate crucial processes such as mood, sleep, and energy. When you eat food, its nutritional content directly impacts how you feel, how you look, and how healthy you are—or are not. That's a lot of power sitting there on your plate, and yet for many of us, it isn't until we are not well or don't have the body or energy or immunity or blood chemistry we desire that it becomes critical to learn how to use that power.

No matter what you are struggling with, your food choices are contributing to that struggle. But your food choices can also contribute to the solution. You are not destined to decline—to lose energy, health, fitness, function, and vitality. It's just the opposite. You have the power to solve your health issues. We all eat, and my heart's desire is to show you how powerful that action can be.

I write prescriptions using food as medicine, and I have spent my entire career learning what specific foods target which specific body systems and health issues. If you want to change something about your body, energy, or health, I'm your girl. I'm not a medical doctor and I don't write prescriptions for medications, but I am a nutritionist and my food prescriptions have been proven to enact real clinical change.

As I have been in the thick of working on this book, I have done a lot of soul searching about why I decided to step out of my comfy-cozy clinic world and move into the world of books and websites and newsletters. I had been sharing my thoughts on our bodies and wellness with those I met face to face, those who were struggling with a variety of health issues behind closed doors. But I didn't feel that went far enough. I have always said that I was thrust into this industry because of my own health crisis. But I think another very important reason that I came out of my clinic and went public with what I know was to create health for you. I have been privileged to walk with my clients through their health crises, and I have learned so much on these journeys that I feel compelled to share that learning with you. Food is such powerful medicine. I not only believe but also know for a fact that food, the right food, can truly heal the body.

But it did start with me and my own health struggles. You see, long before nutritional healing became my profession, it was something I needed to obsess about in order to reclaim my footing on my own slippery slope. I had to work through what food could do for me before I ever had to do it for anyone else. It was a matter of life and death.

MY PATH FROM THE BARN TO THE CLINIC

I was well on my way to vet school when I had to take a medical leave of absence that forced me to learn who I was and what I wanted to become, both personally and professionally. So when I set out to write my first book, *The Fast Metabolism Diet*, I knew that my readers would want to know something about me before considering my advice on weight loss. Many had seen my clients on the red carpet, and because of this, they knew the quality of my sculpting work. Yet, I felt that they needed to know more about my personal credentials: Who am I and how did I learn to *do that*? I told readers about my training in the agricultural industry and animal science, and how I went on to study in many different fields to glean the best of what works from many different traditions.

When I wrote my cookbook, I took it a step further. I wanted readers to know about my culinary experience. Specifically, I wanted them to know that my family has a personal chef . . . and it's me. I'm a mom and I make meals for my kids all day long. When I wrote *The Burn*, I took a slightly different approach to personal disclosure. I wanted readers to understand that many of my clients are not just perfect-seeming celebrities who are already in great shape and just need a little tweaking. I wanted people to understand that in my clinic, during my more than twenty years of experience, I have witnessed firsthand how although people's bodies are not all the same, there's that one commonality—a tendency to get stuck on a plateau; and that searching for the *why* and micro-repairing can unlock the firepower of the metabolism.

Now, with this book, I have a different story to tell, because what I am about to ask you to do, and where I am about to ask you to go, requires something more than information about my training, clinical experience, or even family life. Now, you need to know that when it comes to personal health struggles, I have been there. I have done that. I continue to fight every day. My life is a balancing act between health and health struggles, and without food to keep me in the center of what could be a pretty lethal teeter-totter, I would be lost.

Because this is my fourth book—our fourth book together, for those of you who have been with me from the beginning—I feel as if we have been through so much self-discovery together that you are like a client or a friend. (Welcome, new friends, as well!) We are all on a journey of self-exploration, self-discovery, and self-healing. We have broken bread together, and we have worked on healing some really broken relationships around food. Assuming you are my friend will allow me to be more candid with you and more forthcoming than I have been in any of my previous books.

So let me take a deep breath and give you a little insight into where I come from and why I believe so deeply in the medicinal power of food.

I was born with crazy food, contact, and inhalant allergies. I also have an autoimmune disease called idiopathic thrombocytopenic purpura (ITP). This means I tend to have a very low platelet count because my immune system mistakenly attacks my own platelets. The result is that my blood doesn't clot very well. This can lead to easy bruising and uncontrolled bleeding. Sometimes this condition isn't that serious. Children sometimes develop it and then it goes away. In my case, it is chronic and I will live with it for the rest of my life. When I bleed, it is an emergency, such as when I once had a ruptured ovarian cyst. I found out about the disease when I hemorrhaged during a tonsillectomy when I was seventeen years old.

My mom said I was born running. And even as a child, I never let health issues get in my way. I used to develop lesions on my eyelids and fingers and hands from systemic eczema, and I would buy boxes of Band-Aids and tape up all my fingers and then wear white cotton gloves or my riding gloves over them. The barn was really the only place that felt perfectly normal for a kid to wear gloves all day. When I got back home at night, I would soak my hands in warm water laced with Betadine because the blood and sweat would make the bandages stick to my hands. I also had horrific eczema in the crooks of my arms and on the backs of my knees. When we went to the beach, the salt and sand would aggravate it, causing terrible pain. I would cry and cry the whole way home from the beach, but I would beg my mom to go again when the pain subsided a few days later. This was life with an autoimmune disorder—at least, until I learned how to use food to keep things under control.

Then, when I was twenty-five, I was in a horrific, near-fatal car accident. Because of closed-head trauma, I was an outpatient at the brain injury recovery center for three years and also had to have my entire shoulder rebuilt. I was in a cast from my hip to my thumb, with my thumb out like a hitchhiker for nine weeks, and then my arm casted across my waist for another eight weeks. The accident left me with a central nervous system pain disorder called reflex sympathetic dystrophy syndrome (RSD). I made the mistake of reading my chart once, on which a doctor had written, "One of the worst cases of RSD I've ever seen. Likely to commit suicide." Do you know what it's like to read a note from a doctor saying you are likely to experience so much pain in your life that you will probably off yourself? Let me tell you, it's not fun. But this inspired me to really dive in and study what was happening to me—the why. What were the metabolic pathways involved with a nervous system disorder? That's when I first turned seriously to food and alternative therapies—to ease the pain and protect my psyche.

I could probably turn in my body based on the Lemon Law because I also learned, after two family members and I all had miscarriages within a few weeks of each other, that we were all homozygous for a mutation in the MTHFR (methylenetetrahydrofolate reductase) gene. This is a genetic condition that basically translates to an inability to assimilate folic acid efficiently.

As we all know because of the great work and publicity the March of Dimes has done over the years, folic acid is essential to prevent certain types of birth defects and also to lessen the risk of miscarriage. The March of Dimes slogan is: "Every woman every day," meaning every woman should take a folic acid supplement every day. In my case, this wouldn't be beneficial because my genetics prevent me from utilizing the traditional form of folic acid. This put me at a very high risk of miscarriage, and a much higher risk for having a baby with a spinal defect.

And as if that weren't enough, I also learned that I have something called fragile X syndrome. This is an inherited condition in which the X chromosome is more vulnerable to damage, especially from folic acid deficiency. In extreme cases, this can lead to severe cognitive dysfunction or disabilities, including autism. In my case, it has resulted in a pretty extreme case of dyslexia and ADHD (attention deficit hyperactivity disorder)—things that, at this point in my life, I am actually grateful for because they have helped me to establish priorities and led me to my purpose. Through this, I have created a supportive community. These things were a real struggle when I was younger, but now I've learned to manage them and they also serve as a reminder of why I am here.

Another deep breath is required here because I don't typically share all these things. So, how do I survive with all these health issues? I think a better question is: How have I managed not just to survive but also to *thrive* with them? When I was at the hematologist the other day (I have to see him regularly because of my ITP), he told me, "You know, you really are too healthy to be here. I don't get it. Your labs are beautiful, and yet you have an irreversible genetic bleeding disorder."

"Great," I said. "Then I don't have to come back!"

"I'll see you in four months," he said with a smile. "But I still don't get it."

This kind of visit to the doctor always reminds me to be grateful. Today, my labs are beautiful, and I have food to thank for that. I haven't been on prednisone since I was twenty-one, and I have food to thank for that. I delivered two beautiful and healthy children, and I have food to thank for that. I deal with my RSD without medication, and I have food to thank for that. I wrote three *New York Times* bestsellers despite my learning disabilities. I have a thriving career. I feel good—right here, right now. And I have food to thank for all of it.

I believe I didn't go through all this just so *I* could be healthy. I know that it was so that I could help you. I want you, too, to thank food for how good you feel, how well your health issues have been resolved, and how fully able you are to embrace and live your life. I want you to have the same kinds of successes and triumphs that I have had. We all have bad days, but there can be more good days. Many, many more.

Fortunately for me—and for you, too—I know how to use food to manipulate my own body chemistry to overcome these challenges, genetic and otherwise. I haven't been able to alter my genetic makeup, but I have navigated the expression of my genetic destiny. My health issues do not impact my life the way they "should," according to modern medicine. I don't let them. I do not choose to accept that they are my destiny. I am living proof that I can be healthy, and so can you.

I don't want to go on and on about this. There are enough books out there that tell you how terrible things are. I would rather get to solutions. This is not a book in which we bemoan the state of food in the world, or the obesity rates, or the prevalence of heart disease—or even our own health issues. There are plenty of people already doing that, and we don't need another book like that. Your time is valuable and precious to me, and I have a business to run, kids to raise, and horses to ride. I don't take your time or my time lightly, and I especially don't take lightly the time we have chosen to spend together. That's why this isn't a book based on theory or statistics, or fear of what might happen. This is a book based on food solutions. I know I don't have time to sit around thinking about how bad everything is for me. My medical chart is enough to scare the crap out of me. If I let myself, I could freak out with worry every time I put anything in my mouth, but I'm too busy concentrating on getting my blood levels stable *today* so I can do the work I need to do *today*.

I refuse to live in fear. Our time on this planet is too limited for that. I'd rather live my life in joy, and the fact is that I'm in love with food. I adore food—and you will, too, when you see what it can do for you. I have to say that I am grateful for all those doctors and scientists and gurus who have come before me and clarified what we don't need in our lives—the foods that are killing us or making us fat and addicted. It's just not practical for me to focus on that sort of thing. I need answers, not more things to be afraid of. This book is about turning to food for real results, not banishing foods for fear that they are "bad." I assume if you are reading this book, this kind of thinking isn't practical for you, either. Answers are practical. Solutions are practical. *Food* is practical, and in my world, food is the best form, the safest form, and a remarkably effective form of medicine. It's not to be feared. It is to be embraced.

This is what I want to do for you: I want to sit down with you and find out where you would like to see improvement in your health when your body has gone sideways. Are you concerned about a chronic health issue? Maybe you have chronic indigestion, or constant fatigue. Maybe you have hormonal issues or high cholesterol or depression, or maybe you even have a diagnosis of prediabetes, diabetes, or an autoimmune disease. Every one of these health conditions is a matter of a specific kind of metabolic dysfunction, impaired metabolic pathways; food and natural therapies, therefore, can create the foundation to rebuild lost health. Food is the answer if you want to give your body what it needs to get itself right again.

If you are like my clients—and by that, I mean, if you are a dynamic human being living in a biodiverse world, having multiple positive and not-so-positive health experiences (and I'm thinking you are)—you probably need information on more than one of these issues, so I wrote this book for you. We are going to sit down together, and you are going to tell me your story—I've candidly shared mine and now I want to know yours. Then I'm going to give you a plan. I'll start with the basics—what every healthy person should be doing most of the time—and then we'll look at what you can do, specifically, to target your issues and make them better. I am also committed to creating an active community online, where you can go for support and additional information about all the issues you are working on, including hundreds of additional recipes for the nutritional prescriptions in this book. Find us at www.hayliepomroy.com. We are waiting for you.

Our bodies are stronger and more resilient than we ever imagine. In my body and in the bodies of thousands of my clients over the past twenty years, I have witnessed things that should have been impossible. Health tragedies that felt out of control and people destined for physical decline, but who have reversed and remedied their issues.

Before a lecture, my husband always says, "Let 'er rip, Babe! They didn't come to hear you lecture. They came here because they need your help." This is how I think of you. The formality of a book can get in the way of the relationship between you and me and your quest to find your way back to the health you need, so I am going to do what I do for all of my beloved clients. I am going to give you what I've got, and then we are going to sculpt it and mold it and customize it to end the dysfunctional adaptations happening in your body right now—and restore the perfection that is you when your body has the support it needs.

This is the power of food, and the power of knowledge about what food can do. This is the power of *Fast Metabolism Food Rx*. My own body, my clients, and our community have been the best teachers. It's not just time to eat. It's time to eat to treat.

PART ONE

A Revolutionary Prescription

CHAPTER 1

E + M = H:
An Equation for Health

My health is important, so I learn everything I can about nutrition.
—Louise Hay

When was the last time you ate a tomato? Maybe it was a week ago. Maybe it was today. Maybe you don't like tomatoes and have no interest in eating them. But science is interested in tomatoes. Specifically, science is interested in breaking the tomato down into its component parts, isolating the parts that seem to do some good for human health, and then testing whether they really do or not. It's a fascinating process, but does it translate to anything that will help you decide whether or not to put a tomato on your salad?

One of the things science has figured out about tomatoes is that they contain a phytonutrient called lycopene that gives them their red color. Science has also demonstrated that lycopene in particular seems to have cardioprotective health benefits. Interesting, right? In fact, recently, in 2014, a study was published in *Advanced Nutrition* that compared tomato intake to lycopene supplements (lycopene taken out and isolated and put into a capsule) to see which had a more beneficial effect on markers of cardiovascular disease.[1] And guess who won? The tomato! The study concluded that tomatoes have more positive impact on human health than supplements.

This is all very exciting—and great news. I always love reading about a new study that supports the notion food can influence health. However, what does this information actually have to do with you? The study doesn't tell you what to do with tomatoes. The scientists don't come to your house and consider your life, and advise you about tomatoes. Are you supposed to lay the tomatoes on your chest at night and hope the magic happens? Are you supposed to eat them for every meal for the rest of your life to ensure you won't ever have a heart attack? Or is the occasional tomato enough to benefit you? What is the dosage of tomatoes? And what are the specific benefits you can count on? And furthermore, can you ever really know whether tomatoes, for you as a unique individual with an unprecedented biochemistry, will actually make any difference at all?

What happens in a lab does not (and cannot, by its very nature) possibly predict what will happen when you, with your individual body, metabolism, and circumstances, eat a tomato or any other food. Are you even prone to heart disease? If you are, is your body able to get the lycopene out of the tomato and send it where it needs to go? Can you grab those cardioprotective elements from that tomato in the same way some other random person on the street could or couldn't?

Food can do profound things for you, but you have to have a body that can use it properly to enact those protections and healing compounds. You have to have a body that is set up for creating health out of food. You have to have a metabolism that works. You can deliver a giant pile of 2 x 4s to a building site and they can be the highest quality, most dense, and sturdiest oak available, but if the workers don't show up or have never been trained in how to build a house, that wood is going to sit there and rot. The quality doesn't matter if the house can't get built. Or what if it's a log cabin to be constructed and the only thing delivered were steel beams? That won't help in getting a log cabin built.

It's exactly the same with "power foods." You have to have a body that can take those raw materials and actually make the magic happen. Health is an equation, and it is not as simple as eating a tomato, or taking a pill, or going for a walk, or any other one thing, but it isn't too complicated for us to understand, either.

So what are you struggling with? Is it low energy, premenstrual syndrome (PMS), or menopausal symptoms, irritable bowel syndrome (IBS), indigestion, high cholesterol, or even a chronic disease like diabetes or an autoimmune disorder? No matter what it is, you probably already know you need to do something different. Maybe you have seen a doctor, or maybe you want to try achieving better health on your own, but either way you need a prescription. I'm not talking about a pharmaceutical prescription. I'm talking about a food prescription—one that can have a greater, more lasting, and more restorative effect than anything else you ever do for yourself.

The term for prescription so often used by doctors and pharmacists is Rx, but what "Rx" actually stands for is the Latin word *recipere*, which means "recipe." A food prescription is a recipe for health. The foods you choose and when you eat them can change everything about your energy level, your mood fluctuations, your changing body shape, the numbers on your lab tests like blood pressure and cholesterol, and even the course of chronic diseases that may have already gotten a foothold in your system.

How can food be so powerful? Because food integrates with your body to create health in a powerful way. I like to explain this using an equation so simple that at first it may seem less significant than it actually is: E + M = H. I repeat:

$$E + M = H$$

Here's what it means:

E	+	M	=	H
Eating		Metabolism		Health
Exercise		Metabolic pathways		Homeostasis
Environment		Me		Harmony

- **E is what you eat,** how much you Exercise, and the Environment in which you live, breathe, move, and think. Both eating and exercise create your internal environment, but E is also your external environment, influenced by everything around you, from your family and friends to your job, to what you do with your free time, even to the weather. E is everything you put into your body, everything you do with your body, and everything with which you surround your body.

- **M is your metabolism,** or your rate of converting food into energy. It is also your Metabolic Pathways, which are the many possible roads down which micronutrients (that come from what you eat) travel. Finally, M is the "Me" in the equation—you as an individual, your genetic makeup, your belief systems, your life experiences. This is how your individual body works and what it is doing at any given moment. Your metabolic pathways are the result of biochemical decisions in your body and what they do. For example, you have a metabolic pathway that controls what your body does with sugar. You have one that controls what your body does with hormones. You have another one that controls how your body processes toxins, from substances like medications and pollution. You even have one that translates your thoughts into physical reactions and causes tissues to secrete hormones. All of these influence the M and make you who you are. M is what happens inside you.

- **H is Health.** Health doesn't always mean you are disease free. Instead, it means your body has created a Homeostasis, or internal balance. It means you are living in Harmony with a body that is naturally in a constant state of healthy adaptation or flux. It is the end result of how you combine E with M. It is how you feel right now and how well your body is working. Maximizing the H is what we all hope and strive for, and what we will accomplish with the information in this book's pages.

E + M = H. This equation applies and is working for (or against) you all the time, from your first to your last day on this earth. What science knows is true, even though this knowledge doesn't always trickle down into clinical practice, is that *what you eat and do* (your environment) combined with your *individual metabolism* and *how well your metabolic pathways function* (the "me") determine your health status, your body's ability to maintain homeostasis, and your state of harmony in the present moment.

Although we're talking about equations, I'm not trying to create a teacher-student dynamic. We are on this journey together. Now, the focus is on *your* self-discovery. Together we will explore what the equation means in your life as the formula holds the key to impacting how you feel, the way you look, what your lab reports say, and how healthy you are today and moving forward. Your health depends on two things: E and M. What you do to your body (eating, exercise, and the environment you provide), and what your body is doing to run things (metabolism, metabolic pathways) and be who it is ("me"), creates how well you are able to live (health). Your internal and external environments combined with your individual makeup and the way your body runs directly result in the quality of your health. E + M = H.

When you embrace the implications of E + M = H, you will understand that you have the power to change how your body works—how it feels, how it looks, and how it functions. Depending on what problem you have right now (crushing fatigue, hormonal or digestive issues, metabolic syndrome or diabetes, or autoimmunity), you can use specific food prescriptions to change your internal environment, thereby altering your metabolism in a way that addresses the problem (fills you with energy, balances your hormones, heals your digestion, balances your blood sugar and insulin, or even calms your overactive immune response). Because everyone has a different "M" (metabolism, metabolic pathways, "me") no one "E" (eating plan, exercise, environment) is right for everyone to create health (and homeostasis and harmony). No two metabolisms work in exactly the same way to create a healthy body, and no two bodies are the same. This is why eating on its own cannot create health.

Yet, what you eat profoundly influences your metabolism, which is why metabolic intervention alone (such as with pharmaceuticals) cannot create true health. You need both variables working in concert. The diet industry hasn't embraced this formula yet, and so many people's health would be positively impacted if they would. Instead, they will tell you that E = H. That is, Eating = Health, or even worse, they will tell you to "eat less, exercise more," and that will be the ticket to health. They promote the concept that a particular diet (often one that eliminates a food group, such as carbs or meat, or that slashes calories) will fix everyone's problems. That for some crazy reason, doing less will result in health (or at least weight loss).

We hear a lot of crazy health rumors. Maybe you've heard that if you eat an apple a day, you will keep the doctor away. That if you eat chia seeds and raw cacao, and breathe out of alternating nostrils, you can cure every disease you've ever had. They can have valid effects, but until you repair your metabolic pathways using food strategically, these health strategies aren't going to do much for you. (Although I have to admit, raw cacao brings me joy!) What good is the energy in an apple if you can't metabolize the sugar? What good are the nutrients in chia seeds or raw cacao if you can't absorb them? What good is the stress-reducing power of alternate-nostril breathing if your body isn't recognizing the relaxation response? Fix the pathways first. Then you can actually benefit from that apple and the many other "super foods" and strategies that science says can impact your risk of heart disease, cancer, Alzheimer's, advanced aging, and other chronic diseases.

Many doctors, and for sure drug companies, are more likely to see the formula like this: M = H. That is, metabolism, or what your body is or isn't doing, determines your health. Your lab reports say your body is pooling cholesterol in the blood, your LDLs are high; this means you are not metabolizing cholesterol, and many doctors are likely to say that to change those numbers, you need a statin drug. Many physicians may even believe it has nothing to do with what you eat. Doctors often say (even to me) that a certain health problem is not related in any way to diet—that it is a genetic or age-related problem. Have you ever been told (or just believed) that you will get diabetes, that you will probably get heart disease because it runs in your family, that you will have early-onset menopause because your mother did, or that you come from a long line of individuals with depression and therefore that is your destiny? You might possess those genes, but it is the alteration in the metabolic pathways that stimulates the expression of them. I've had healthy debates with many doctors who tell me that the issue for the client we are talking about has nothing to do with food. I'm surprised every time. What your metabolism does is directly impacted by the food you eat, how and when you eat it, and in what combination you eat it with other nutrients. How is this not obvious to everyone? E can't = H and M can't = H. You need both E and M to achieve health. E + M = H.

In my practice, I encourage a high degree of self-study. Self-discovery, if you will. I want you to become absorbed in what your metabolism is doing by noticing how you feel and react to the foods you eat. Don't worry. You're mine now, and we will explore *you* together. Let's look at the things you commonly do—even the thoughts you think, the sleep you are or are not having, and the deep desires you have for your health. I want us to look at your current E (eating, environment, exercise) and what we can define about your M (metabolism), so that we can recognize how they are affecting your H. I need you to become a little bit self-centered on your own behalf, but don't worry; I will be standing next to you evaluating that reflection in the mirror.

This may go against everything you think you are supposed to do and be. You may feel selfish, but trust me—this kind of self-examination is the foundation for health and the ultimate key to being there for everyone else. Just imagine that I am sitting across the desk from you, saying, "Welcome to my office. I am so excited to get to know you. Tell me all about yourself. How do you feel? What has changed recently? What's bothering you? What is your body doing? How do you wish you felt? How is your chemistry? What are your bowel movements, libido, energy, and sleep like? How is your immune system? Your blood sugars? What are you doing to and for your body?" and of course, "What do you crave? And what are you eating?"

Your answers to these questions are clues to your metabolism and your metabolic pathways and how they interact with what you eat. Health is not contained in a generic, one-size-fits-all list of good foods and bad foods, or foods to add and foods to subtract. People are not generic, one-size-fits-all carbon copies of each other. Thank God. Yawn. How boring would that be? Foods (and everything else you do) are the E, but to change your health, the nature of what happens to what you eat depends on the action of your individual metabolism.

So who are you? How are you feeling? What is your metabolism doing today? What is your body revealing to you about your unique metabolism that can give you clues about what to eat? Only when we look at who you are, where you have been, where you want to go, and what your health desires are—in other words, what your metabolism is doing—only then can you go to the grocery store and know what to buy to create meaningful health change. Only then can you know what to make for dinner to give you energy, or balance your hormones, or make you feel happier today—or help you metabolize cholesterol and balance your blood sugars and control your autoimmune disease. The real key to health is to be able to empower the body and purposefully manipulate *what your unique body does with the particular foods you eat*. When you can do that, then you suddenly have all the power, sitting right there on your plate.

EATING

We all have to eat. Wouldn't it be amazing, then, if this thing we have to do each day could create an abundance of health? The E is about eating food, exercising your body, and manipulating your environment, but it is most powerfully controlled by your food choices.

To effect any kind of metabolic change—to take back control of the way your body adapts to its environment, to repair broken pathways, to speed up sluggish pathways, and to reopen ones that have shut down—you have to change what you are doing. My favorite way to do that is with food, or with your D.I.E.T. In my world, D.I.E.T. is an abbreviation for: "Did I Eat Today?"

The most important question you can ask yourself is, "Did I Eat Today?" To me, D.I.E.T. has nothing to do with doing without. It has nothing to do with deprivation.

- Did I eat today for more energy?

- Did I eat today to feel good all day long?

- Did I eat today to balance my hormones?

- Did I eat today for better skin, hair, and nails?

- Did I eat today to stimulate my libido?

- Did I eat today to scavenge cholesterol from my blood?

- Did I eat today to lower my triglycerides?

- Did I eat today to feel more joy?

- Did I eat today to reverse my autoimmune disease?

- Did I eat today to solve my blood sugar issues?

Whatever your goals, whatever it is you want for your body and your health, ask yourself: Did you eat today to accomplish that goal? Food is *essential for metabolic repair*. To achieve the results you want, the energy you crave, the body you desire, and the health you dream about, you cannot fear food. You cannot avoid food. You must embrace food. You must have a love affair with food because of all it can do for you. You must continually ask yourself: Did I Eat Today? And together, we are going to discover and define how to eat to repair the metabolic adaptation your body is making and create a perfect equation for your health.

My answer to your health issues will never be, "You should eat less." There is no minus sign in E + M = H. Even if weight loss is your goal and you need to lose 100 pounds, eating less is never the answer. Food—not the lack of it—is always the way to address a metabolism that is adapting to your current environment in a way you don't like. But you have to add food to your metabolism to get a result.

What, how, and when you eat will be unique to your circumstances and the changes you are attempting to evoke. This is using food as medicine. You will be eating the foods that invoke the metabolic solutions to your problems. But before we get to the M and what that's all about—even before I give you a single dietary prescription—what I want you to understand is that food must be a priority. Going without food is never going to solve your problem.

In my family, food is a big deal. I mean a Big Deal. The other day, my friend was taking my kids to school, and when I walked into the kitchen just after they left, I saw that breakfast was still sitting on the table. I immediately called my son.

"Get back here and eat your breakfast," I said.

"But Mom, I'll be late!" he said.

"I don't care."

"I'll get Saturday detention if I'm late!"

"I don't care. You turn around and you get back here, and you eat breakfast," I said.

And that was that.

A client of mine is forty-three years old and has multiple health issues we are working to resolve. Weight gain was one result of her metabolism and metabolic pathways going out of balance. Since we've been working together, she's lost 42 pounds and has another 35 to go. When she started, she was always looking at the end goal. She told me that she'll never forget how, when she first came into my office, she kept asking about getting to her goal weight, and I didn't want to talk about that. I said, "We'll talk about your goal weight later. Right now, let's just get you healthy. Let's check off the list of health issues as a priority, and the weight will come along." She remembers asking,

"But what are we going to set as a goal weight?"

And I just said, "We'll negotiate that, but let's see what your body tells us first."

She said this was the first time she realized what she was actually trying to do for herself wasn't really about losing weight. It was about creating a different kind of relationship with food and finally becoming healthy. She said this was a concept that had been completely unfamiliar to her. She'd been in deprivation mode, but never truly thinking about real nourishment. She had not realized the power of food.

Another friend has a son dealing with some health issues (which I will keep private), and as he struggled with his health, he said that for the first time he could feel the connection between how he felt and how he was eating. He's on some powerful medications, but he has also revamped his diet to contain mostly whole foods in conjunction with a supplement regimen. All the side effects of his medications have faded and he's feeling great. This is when he noticed that his girlfriend purchased food based strictly on price. "She eats the most horrible processed foods because she can get them on sale three for a dollar," he said. "I used to do that! And now I would never! I can't imagine ever going back to eating that way. I would feel terrible!"

Of course, food isn't just the answer. It can also be the problem, not because of its presence but because of its absence (dieting, fasting, scarcity) and because of its quality. We live in a time and place when we have more cheap, artificial food available to us than ever before, and yet we often fear food, starve ourselves, or obsess about it in unhealthy ways—like eliminating entire food groups or freaking out if we think we ate the wrong thing.

When you eat fake food, processed food, or low-quality food, though, you inadvertently create an internal environment (E) that will force your body to adapt (M) in ways you might not like. I'll talk more about this in the next chapter, but for now let's just say that real, whole food is the only kind of food I recommend. Really, it is the only thing that should be called food.

Unfortunately, it isn't as easy to get as the fake stuff, yet it should be. The other day I was in a grocery store, and I saw a big sign over a very small section of one aisle. It said: *HEALTHY FOOD*. I stopped and stared. Am I the only one who thinks it is totally asinine that there's a "healthy" section in the grocery store? That just half of one aisle contains foods officially deemed "healthy"? If that half an aisle has what's healthy, what is in the rest of the store? What is that store telling you about its products? It tells me, in big bold letters, that if you eat here, you will be unhealthy. Weird marketing, I think.

In the attempt to solicit business from people who are trying to live healthy lives, that are suffering from metabolic disorders such as fatigue, diabetes, autoimmunity, and high cholesterol and the like, the manufacturers of these foods are flat-out saying, "We manufacture two kinds of foods. One kind is healthy." Let's hope they are not participating in false advertising, and that one kind actually is healthy. If I served you food that was rotten, would you eat it? If I served you food with maggots in it, would you eat it? Never mind that maggots are more nutritionally dense than many of the food additives in the grocery store. We don't eat maggots in our culture, and if you came to my home and I served you maggots, I hope you would be offended. And yet we are eating pesticides and even paint thinner. We are feeding our children carcinogens and neurotoxins, and most people don't even think about it. Many don't even know about it—at least not how poisonous it truly is to have these substances as part of our diet.

We are eating food that is not good for us, sometimes with the full knowledge that it is not good for us. We are eating food that has been proved over and over and over again to cause diseases such as obesity and diabetes and heart disease and cancer. The information is out there. Why aren't we getting it? Why is this "food" ending up on all our plates? Quite frankly, why is it allowed to be sold?

So, let's make eating a priority. Let's explore strategic ways to employ real, delicious food to heal our bodies. If you can shift your thinking so that healthy food is the only food acceptable for you and your family, then you have taken a giant step in the right direction. Don't worry, I'm going to show you how.

You'll also learn that food can do even more for you. Food can make specific changes in your metabolism, which can usher in exacting alterations to your health. My clients often come to me with specific issues. They want to fix how they feel, or how they look, or address the lab reports that reveal the onset of a health issue. When my clients ask me questions about what they should do, my answer is always E + M = H, and it always begins: "You should be eating. . . ."

YOU: "How do I get more energy?"

ME: "You should be eating . . ."

YOU: "Why can't I exercise like I used to? I get so tired."

ME: "You should be eating . . ."

YOU: "What can I do about my terrible PMS?"

ME: "You should be eating . . ."

YOU: "What can I do about my high cholesterol?"

ME: "You should be eating . . ."

YOU: "My doctor said I'm prediabetic. What do I do?"

ME: "You should be eating . . ."

YOU: "What about my constant hunger?"

ME: "You should be eating . . ."

YOU: "Is there any way to prevent the chronic disease so many people in my family get?"

ME: "Yes! You should be eating . . ."

People on my forums are constantly sharing stories about their health struggles and their successes. Some have lagging energy or they just don't feel good, even though their doctors can't find anything wrong. Some struggle with out-of-control weight gain or body-shape changes they don't understand. Some have been diagnosed with something like diabetes, or prediabetes, or an autoimmune disease, or high cholesterol, or high blood pressure, or heart disease. Some are depressed, or having panic attacks. But as different as they are as individuals, they all want to know the same thing: *What should I do? What should I do that is unique to me and my issues?*

You should be eating to balance the equation so you can repair the metabolism and regain health.

METABOLISM

Metabolism affects every single aspect of your life, from your bones, hair, skin, nails, tendons, and ligaments to your moods, immune system function, stress hormone production, cholesterol metabolism, libido, memory, and cognition. Metabolism is the big-picture process of how your body takes things in and transforms them for energy, rebuilding, and repairing. Your metabolism is the way your unique body adapts to your unique environment. It is what your body does with the food you eat. To do anything at all, your body must take in food and process it, extracting what it needs and eliminating what it doesn't. Then it must use what it has extracted to do the work of repairing, rebuilding, and replenishing *you*. There are many complex biochemical mechanisms by which this works, and it's happening inside you all the time.

The word *metabolism* comes from the Greek word *metabolismos*, which means "to change." The very concept is dynamic, not static. If your environment shifts (such as with a dietary change or a toxic exposure, or from stress in your life, or because you need to lift something heavy or run fast, or you miss sleep, or even because the way you feel about your life changes), your metabolism will change so you can adapt. The metabolism is agile, and that's good news for you, because that means you can learn how to manipulate your metabolism. When you change your metabolism, you can potentially change almost anything about how your body works. All you have to do is listen to what your body is telling you, and then supply your body with strategic micronutrients—the ones it needs to accomplish the necessary work.

The metabolism works in some basic ways for everyone, but it is also highly individual to the person. The way the body reacts to food doesn't happen the same way in any two people. You cannot tell me that the sandwich my little ninety-year-old, 92-pound grandmother eats for lunch does the same thing in her body that the sandwich a twenty-five-year-old, 250-pound weightlifter eats does in his body. My grandmother and our big, buff bodybuilder have completely different metabolisms, and therefore, they have completely different nutritional needs if they both want to be healthy.

The foods you eat and the energy they contain determine what your metabolism does. Your body looks at what it's got to work with and then it goes to work. The metabolism is the mechanism by which your body gets its jobs done. Know yourself, and you will know your metabolism—and that is how you will know what to eat. You can't tell me that somebody with heart disease should be eating the same way as somebody with diabetes, or that somebody with severe depression should be eating the same way as somebody who wants to get a better time on the next run or wishes to spice things up in the bedroom. You can put the best fuel in the world in your car, but it won't matter if the engine is broken—or if you're trying to put jet fuel into your Honda. The fuel is what you eat. The engine is your metabolism. The car's performance is your health. Even an engine in tip-top shape can be destroyed by the wrong fuel.

WHAT ARE METABOLIC PATHWAYS?

If the metabolism is an engine, the metabolic pathways are the moving parts that make the engine work—the pistons and the crankshaft and the rods. They are the mechanisms by which the metabolism works—the individual parts that help convert food into energy, movement, and change. Metabolism pathways transform some things into other things, making them bioactive and therefore useful to the body. They involve a series of chemical reactions in the body and their sum total equals the metabolism.

Metabolic pathways determine the life cycle of a hormone or a nutrient. They influence the formation and maturation of blood cells or immune cells. They determine how we store or burn blood sugar, and whether it gets sent to the brain or muscle or into fat cells. A metabolic pathway's action is determined by what enzymes are secreted, what hormones are secreted, whether the liver makes the hormone bioactive, whether the receptor site receives the hormone, and a million other variables. Every one of these actions is nutrient dependent and therefore is influenced by the food you take in and what you do with that food metabolically. How you feel or when you eat can alter the metabolic pathways the nutrients that you extract end up taking.

Metabolic disorders like diabetes or elevated cholesterol are basically breakdowns, diversions, or dysfunctions in any of hundreds of metabolic pathways (and for every metabolic pathway science has been able to define, there are probably hundreds more we don't know about yet or haven't defined). This isn't just something nutritionists or alternative-medicine doctors believe. This is what governmental organizations state—organizations like the National Institutes of Health and the National Institute of Diabetes and Digestive and Kidney Diseases, which calls diabetes and obesity "metabolic disorders";[2] and organizations like the National Heart, Lung, and Blood Institute that list abdominal obesity, high triglycerides (a type of fat found in the blood), low HDL ("good") cholesterol levels, high blood pressure, and high fasting blood sugar as "metabolic risk factors."[3] Science knows that the metabolism is directly linked to obesity, that excess body fat changes the metabolism and the way it reacts to food,[4] and that substances that manipulate the metabolism,[5] including dietary alterations,[6] directly affect physical performance.

But these things don't act in isolation from each other. The body is a complex, living organism and changes in the metabolism set off a complex cascade of changes throughout the metabolic pathways, impacting fitness levels, performance, mood, fat accumulation, body shape, and the chronic diseases your body could eventually develop. For example, there is a metabolic pathway that allows the liver to make hormones bioactive. The ones we don't need—excess hormones—are converted into bile salts. If your body isn't converting estrogen into bile salts, which are then released into the gastrointestinal (GI) tract to break down fat, you will have too much estrogen in your body, which can result in hot flashes. If your body isn't making enough of the hormones you need, or the receptor sites aren't receiving the hormones, then your body may expand the fat cells, which can produce their own estrogen, resulting in hormone-based weight gain.

To get your body bio-adapting to a healthier environment, you need to repair the specific metabolic pathways that aren't working the way they should be in your system. If we fix the metabolism, can we actually eliminate the diseases and other issues of the metabolism? I believe we can—with the right food prescription. It's the best way to address a system with this many complex moving parts. It all goes back to E + M = H. Everything I do to reverse metabolic dysfunction is based on this equation, which works even as it is applied to the amazing diversity of metabolic adaptation happening inside you.

HEALTH

What is health? For you, it might be something different from what is health for anyone else in the world. Is it being fit and free of disease? Is health feeling balanced, or having energy, or getting down to a weight that doesn't burden you? Or is it getting your chronic conditions manageable again?

Whenever a new client comes into my office, one of the first things we do is sit down together and make a Health Wish List. This is a list of everything the client would like to happen. The first things my clients usually mention are that they want to change the number on the scale, and/or they want to change the progression of a chronic disease they have been diagnosed with. I think those goals are too narrow. Why limit yourself to a diagnosis or a number on the scale, or that one, most pressing symptom? I want you to dream big. Think of everything you want for your body. And this can be an ongoing list. You can check things off as you achieve them, and you can always add more. In fact, I encourage you to add more, as you learn more and get to know this process better. I always encourage my clients to go further. Below is a sampling of some of the items my clients have come up with for their own Health Wish Lists. Check the ones that you want on your list, then try to add ten more items at the end of this list that mean something to you.

- ☐ I want more energy.
- ☐ I want to feel good all day long.
- ☐ I want to get rid of my mid-afternoon slump.
- ☐ I want to sleep better.
- ☐ I want to want to have sex!
- ☐ I want to get some of this fat off my hips.
- ☐ I want to banish the back fat!
- ☐ I want to reduce the cellulite on my thighs.
- ☐ I want to get rid of my double chin.

- ☐ I want better, clearer skin.
- ☐ I want to get rid of my wrinkles.
- ☐ I want to get the sag out of my upper arms.
- ☐ I want to stop being constipated.
- ☐ I want to get rid of my indigestion.
- ☐ I want to lower my cholesterol.
- ☐ I want to feel happier.
- ☐ I want to get rid of my anxiety.
- ☐ I want to reverse my autoimmune disease.
- ☐ I want to solve my blood sugar issues.
- ☐ I no longer want to have diabetes!
- ☐ _____
- ☐ _____
- ☐ _____
- ☐ _____
- ☐ _____
- ☐ _____
- ☐ _____
- ☐ _____
- ☐ _____
- ☐ _____

This is just a small sampling. Your list can be much more detailed, much more inclusive, much longer. Actually write it down. Include everything! Dream big. And then recognize something very important: Everything you eat influences the possibility that every single thing on your wish list will come true—or will only remain a dream. This book will guide you toward those areas you desire the most, with solutions to help you achieve your dreams; and in the last chapter, you will find a quiz to help further refine your focus. On my website, www.hayliepomroy.com, you'll find an even more comprehensive digital quiz to help you decide which goals to achieve first, along with hundreds of additional recipes to make your nutritional prescription (which you will receive as you work through this book) exciting and delicious. I have the tools to help guide you, but what you want to achieve and the choice to reclaim the power to achieve it are right there in your hands.

CHAPTER 2

Is It Disease or Metabolic Adaptation?

Inside each of us are two wolves. One is evil. One is good. . . . Which wolf wins? The one you feed.

—Adapted from a Cherokee story, source unknown

Have you ever stood in front of a mirror and asked: *Who are you and what have you done with my body?*

If you don't recognize your face because of its dark circles or new wrinkles or sudden sagging, or if you try to pull up your jeans over your newly larger stomach or hips, or if you've just gotten that look (or even that diagnosis) from your doctor, you may be wondering how you got here. Is this really you? How did this happen? *Is this your body?* And does what you see make you feel uneasy?

Assuming we can bank on the fact that you were probably not abducted by aliens, what's going on? Where did your energy go? Where did your body go? Where did your health go? Where did *you* go? Many of my clients ask me, "How the hell did I get here?"

My answer is always the same, no matter the issue, no matter the degree of change: You got here on purpose. You have a very smart body. Brilliant, even. It knows how to change when its environment changes to preserve your health as well as it can. It knows how to change because of the M in E + M = H. Your body does what it must do in the face of adversity to keep you alive.

Maybe it started with fatigue. You can barely drag yourself out of bed in the morning, or you can't stay awake in the afternoon. Maybe one day you were you, fit and healthy and full of vitality, and then suddenly you were that other person—that strange tired, pale, bloated person with that totally different body and these unexpected health issues. You used to want to have sex all the time and now, well . . . wouldn't it be nicer just to sleep? You used to love exercise, but now it just seems like too much effort. *Who are you?* Maybe you never thought you'd be the person who gave up on exercise. Maybe you have hot flashes, or your hair is falling out, or your digestion reacts to almost everything you eat, or your cholesterol is pooling in your blood, or your doctor has told you that you have a chronic disease, or that you are at serious risk for something like diabetes or heart disease. Maybe it started with allergies or dark circles under your eyes, but now you have arthritis or lupus. Maybe it's chronic pain, or wonky hormones, or out-of-control blood sugar, or maybe you just can't get a good night's sleep.

Extreme fatigue, loss of sex drive, or a decrease in your ability to exercise may not have been part of your game plan, but you are experiencing it right now for a good reason. The seemingly sudden appearance of belly fat or arm flab or wrinkles or a general widening of your entire silhouette might not have been your intention, but your body has changed in an effort to save you from a much worse fate. Disease was most certainly not one of your goals for your life, but what we call disease is actually a calculated response to your environment that has kept you in survival mode. You are where you are right now because the shape of your body and the state of your health are direct reflections of your body's higher purpose: survival.

Here's an analogy I use with my clients. To be financially solvent, you have to have more money coming in than going out. You have to make more than you spend. If you are bringing in more than you are putting out, you can build up your savings account so you have resources for when you really need them, and you won't have to carry a credit card balance and pay interest on the outstanding balance.

This process of income and expenditures, savings and credit, is like your metabolism. Building a savings account is like creating lean muscle, dense bones, and nutrient stores. When your income is greater—when you are giving your body all the nutrients it needs to do its work—you can build these up to get you through the rough times, such as when you are under a lot of stress or don't have access to enough good food. When your income is lessened because you got laid off or went on vacation, you can operate pretty darn well, assuming you have savings to dip into. But what if you don't go back to work for weeks, months, years? You will run through your savings and build up credit card debt, and then when you get to the end of your resources and have to start paying everybody back, you are in serious trouble.

When this happens physiologically, the way your body dips into its savings is to start scavenging nutrients from nonessential biological functions like hair and nail growth. Next, it might start pulling minerals from bones and protein from muscles. You might still look great if you've got strong healthy hair and nails, dense bones, and lots of lean muscle tissue to work with, but eventually it's going to show.

And if you keep going, it's going to start hurting more than your vanity. Your body will accumulate an uneasiness—a dis-ease. It may not be diagnosable at first. Your bones will get more porous. You will lose muscle mass. Your blood chemistry will go off. But at some point, despite your body's very best efforts, you will get sick. You might think your body has betrayed you, but in reality it is doing the very best it can to sustain you. It has had no choice but to find a temporary measure to build up your resources.

Let's take a moment to consider what this chronic discomfort to your body consists of—what chronic disease really is. You may already have a diagnosis, or you may not have one, but most of my clients are headed in that direction when they first come to see me and here's why: Their bodies have been talking, but those clients haven't been listening, and so their bodies have struggled along without guidance and kept them alive despite everything that was happening to them.

This is the heart and soul of this book: If you have a chronic disease, like depression or an autoimmune disorder or metabolic syndrome or diabetes, your metabolism is working as well as it can to help you survive under less than ideal conditions. If you don't have a chronic disease, your body may be warning you that one is in your future if you don't make some changes.

Chronic diseases can compromise the quality of your life. They can be difficult to cure, and they can take over your identity. Yet, you can escape that fate, climb out of the hole you are in right now; your life can be something much better, lighter, freer, healthier, and more beautiful than you realize right now. You can do it with food. A food prescription can help restore a more conducive environment for healing so that you can thrive again.

An imbalance in metabolic pathways is at the crux of all chronic disease.

The metabolism is nutrient dependent. Guess what has zero nutrient value? Drugs. Guess what has exactly the micronutrients your body needs to repair the metabolism? Food! In most cases, outside of surgery: *Food is the only way to repair chronic disease.*

I *WISH* DRUGS CURED CHRONIC DISEASE

Guess who is studying metabolic pathways more closely than anyone else? Pharmaceutical companies. Companies in this multi-billion-dollar industry take all the knowledge they have and continue to gain about what is going wrong in the metabolic pathways, and they use that valuable information to create a pharmaceutical gag order. You don't get a solution or a cure. You get a temporary fix of your symptoms, and that's it. That's because the parties with the drugs who most effectively muffle the symptoms of chronic diseases is the party who "wins."

But you don't win. When you go off the medication, the symptoms come back because the disease is still there. Cortisone for skin issues, Cox inhibitors and NSAIDS for pain, SSRIs for mood problems—all muffle the sound of your body calling out to you that something needs to change.

And it doesn't get you healthy. To get you healthy, we need to take it a step further. Everybody agrees that the metabolic pathways are nutrient dependent, yet those nutrients come from one place and one place only: food. There can be a lot of value in medications; I'm not saying there isn't. But one value no medication has is nutrient value.

This is important to understand if you have a chronic disease or are at risk of developing one. If your metabolism has taken a left turn when it should have taken a right one, and you are metabolically adapting in ways that affect your energy or body shape, chronic disease is probably in your future if you don't change something. Unfortunately, chronic disease is the ultimate outcome for most Americans, and it is also avoidable, so I want you to understand what it is. Whether it is in your present or possibly in your future, *know thy enemy.*

There is a rubric that the medical community uses to define chronic disease. Let's look at that, so we can all be on the same page when we talk about what we can do about it. A disease is considered chronic if:

1. **It doesn't heal by itself.** If you have diabetes or multiple sclerosis or high cholesterol, it's not just going to go away suddenly one day without your doing anything about it.

2. **It grows worse over time.** If you have heart disease, for example, it's gradually going to get worse, rather than better, if you don't intervene. The more your heart function is compromised, the less able your body is to function overall with efficiency, which further compromises heart function. It's a downward spiral.

3. **It does not have a single cause.** Why does somebody become obese or develop an anxiety disorder or get irritable bowel syndrome? It's not exclusively due to one thing. It's not calories, or being sedentary, or one particular stress factor like a job, or high fructose corn syrup, or a polluted environment—each of these things can contribute to the issue.

4. **It creates a complex symptom profile.** Let's say you suffer from clinical depression. Feeling sad certainly isn't the only symptom. You might also be low on energy. You might have trouble sleeping, or waking up. You might have periods of high-intensity emotion and periods of flat affect. You might feel sad some of the time, or all of the time, or only during certain times. Maybe you are affected seasonally, or maybe your depression seems random. You might also have muscle aches or joint pain or chronic headaches.

These four anchors form the rubric by which chronic disease is diagnosed. Considering the nature of this list, you can understand why no single pill will cure a chronic condition. It is common for an individual dealing with chronic disease to be on ten to fourteen pills before he or she ever reaches the Medicare system. I wish that one pill could fix chronic disease, and that this magic pill was affordable and on the market. Science, the medical community, and even the pharmaceutical companies agree that this magic pill doesn't exist, which is why I've dedicated my life's work to repairing the metabolic pathways that contribute to the metabolic risk factors of chronic disease.

For example, in a statement released by the American Heart Association and the National Heart, Lung, and Blood Institute (NHLBI), there are five metabolic risk factors for heart disease:[7]

1. A large waistline, abdominal obesity, or excess belly fat

2. Elevated triglycerides

3. Low HDL cholesterol (what we call the "good" cholesterol because it helps remove LDL, or "bad," cholesterol from your arteries)

4. High blood pressure

5. High fasting blood sugar

Those symptoms cover a lot of ground. The NHLBI then goes on to explain that medication *does not alleviate these risk factors.* Not one of them. Medication might lower your cholesterol or blood pressure while you are on it, but as soon as you go off it, your cholesterol or blood pressure will go back up. Medication might correct your fasting blood sugar or your high triglycerides, but as soon as you go off it, that goes back up, too. The risk factor is still there, even if it's not showing up on a lab test.

You have not changed the reason the blood lipids are pooling in the blood. You haven't changed the reason your blood pressure is high. If you take medication for depression or anxiety, the medication doesn't cure or reverse the disease. If you take medication for chronic indigestion, the medication doesn't cure or reverse that disease, either. If medication did these things, then you could stop taking it and you would be okay. But you won't be.

Do you know how effective a drug has to be to receive official approval? It has to have 33 percent efficacy. That means it only has to work one-third of the time. Last time I checked, that is a failing grade everywhere but in baseball. Sometimes medications are absolutely necessary; if you need them, you should take them for as long as you need them. Medications can be quite effective in fighting and killing bacteria—and a few generations ago, that was a huge leap in medicine. They are also good for pain relief in the event of an acute trauma, like a broken bone. Treating a chronic disease is an entirely different problem, however, and modern medicine just isn't very good at it. The drugs that work so well for acute problems simply don't work well for chronic problems—and again, they certainly don't cure them.

But food? Food is an entirely different story. Remember that your body is constantly adapting to its internal environment. You can invoke real change with food because food delivers the micronutrients that the metabolic pathways depend on to function correctly. Without food, you will die. With it, you can deliver strategic and targeted micronutrients to invoke change. Food allows you to survive, but if you use it as medicine, you can thrive.

Food can also help medications work better. If you ever need a medication for crisis intervention, I want to help ensure that you are one of the 33 percent for which that medication works. The best way to do that is to have the healthiest body possible, and for you to be on the least amount of daily medication possible. I want your body so clean that the medication you need can work in the most profound way.

Did you know multi-drug interactions are one of the leading causes of a drug's not being effective, and that 70 percent of our population is on a pharmaceutical right now? Among those eligible for Medicare, 90 percent are on five or more medications! And guess what the most commonly prescribed medications are in this country today? They are called P.A.N.I.C. meds. These are medications for pain (P), anxiety (A), nausea (N), inflammation (I), and constipation (C).

Every single one of those P.A.N.I.C. conditions, including pain, can be supported with the targeted use of food, but that's not the prescription you are likely to get from your doctor. It is what you will get from me, though. Name one other prescription in the world besides food that is noninvasive, inexpensive, and can actually reverse the disease process. There is not a medication on the market that can do for you what food can do—and what food has done for centuries. For example, I have witnessed food reverse digestive issues like acid reflux, not just suppress them. I have seen food reverse diabetes, not temporarily manipulate insulin the way medication does. I have seen food return cholesterol and lipid levels back to normal, not temporarily blunt blood cholesterol the way medication does.

In my own body, food became my drug of choice after living on 60 mg daily of a powerful steroid called prednisone; that was after trying and reacting (sometimes violently) to naltrexone, methotrexate, gabapentin, imuran, dexmathasone, and many other drugs used off-label as doctors tried to alleviate my life-threatening symptoms. Sure, those drugs invoked some changes. One of those changes was anaphylaxis. But nothing reversed my condition and maintained health the way food does and continues to do in my life every single day.

According to the Centers for Disease Control and Prevention (CDC), chronic diseases are the leading cause of death and disability in the United States.* These include diseases and conditions like heart disease, stroke, cancer, diabetes, obesity, and arthritis. Also according to the CDC, as of 2012, about half of all adults in the United States have one or more chronic health conditions, and about one-fourth of us have two or more chronic health problems.

We also know that these diseases cost us millions. According to the CDC, 86 percent of the country's health-care costs are for treating chronic diseases.† Check out this sampling of chronic disease costs in recent years, just to give you an idea of the numbers we're talking about:

Heart disease and stroke cost about $315 billion in 2010.

Diabetes cost about $245 billion per year in 2012.

Alzheimer's disease cost $148 billion in 2007.

Obesity cost $147 billion in 2008.

---

* Centers for Disease Control and Prevention, "Chronic Diseases and Health Promotion," CDC posting, July 2015, http://www.cdc.gov/chronicdisease/overview/.
† Ibid.

I'm not the only example, of course. A client comes to mind who had a doctor who started her on a diabetes medication called Byetta, which is sometimes used for appetite control. Because the appetite for sugar is important to control from a diabetic perspective, doctors often like to piggyback this medication on another diabetes medication called metformin. In this particular client, Byetta killed her appetite so thoroughly that she went for long periods without eating. But fasting can cause blood sugar to rise. There is a test that measures how well blood sugar and insulin have cooperated in the body and balanced each other, correlating to blood sugar levels over the past two to three months, called hemoglobin A1C. I've seen some clients whose test numbers rise dangerously high when they go for long periods without eating, and as I monitored her, I watched her numbers go up and up and up.

"You need to talk to your doctor," I told her. "I don't think the Byetta and the metformin are the right mix for you."

When she talked to her doctor, however, he said, "No, I really like the way this drug works when coupled with metformin."

This is a case of a doctor applying a generic scenario to an individual patient. In many people, this drug combination works just fine. In her, however, it was a disaster. She needed an intervention, so I went with her to the doctor and I brought the chart. I showed the doctor her fasting blood sugar before Byetta; and in a big red pen, I circled the start date of the drug, and I showed him how the fasting blood sugar had risen significantly. "She seems to have the opposite reaction you normally see with Byetta," I said.

Now this is a very good doctor and he listened to us. He knows a lot. "Wow," he said. "I haven't seen this in my practice before. Let's take you off the Byetta and see what happens." She went off it, and sure enough, her fasting blood sugar levels and other tests that show blood sugar and insulin stability improved. She also regained her appetite just enough that she remembered to eat breakfast regularly in the morning—and in my opinion, that's what really made the difference.

METABOLIC ADAPTATION: A STRESS RESPONSE TO AVOID DISEASE

Let's back up now and look at how all this gets started in your body.

Metabolic adaptation is the way your metabolic pathways adapt to your current environment, both inside and out. The pathways of metabolic adaptation are reactive, responsive, directive, and prescriptive. They tell your body things like:

Hey, liver, we're burning too much energy. Absorb more sugar, we're going to need that energy later!

Hey, bones, we're getting banged around a lot here. Remodel yourselves to be stronger!

Digestion, hold off for a bit—things are getting dicey and we need to conserve resources.

Fat cells, you're good at making estrogen and we can use some more. Make more estrogen, will you?

When it comes right down to it, metabolic adaptation occurs because of stress. Every stressor, whether physical (a marathon, a food binge, an illness) or mental (a big test, a relationship problem, work pressure), and whether the stress feels negative (a virus, a divorce, no downtime) or positive (graduation, a new love, a wedding), changes the body's internal environment. That creates a reason for your metabolism to adapt. Your body is constantly reacting to stress and metabolically adapting to accommodate it.

Stress has a bad reputation, but I want to emphasize that stress is not necessarily a bad thing.[8] We place stress on a door to shut it, and shutting the door keeps the rain and the robbers out. We place stress on our muscles during a workout to lay down healthy muscle tissue. We place stress on our hearts to increase cardiovascular health. We place stress on our digestive system when we eat food, so that it can excrete the right enzymes for digestion. But stress can also go too far.

In a recent study on metabolic adaptation, rats experiencing an acute injury showed dramatic physical changes within six to forty-eight hours following that injury, including a rapid decrease in the size of the thymus, spleen, lymph glands, and liver; they experienced a disappearance of fat tissue, loss of muscle tone, decreased body temperature, and erosions in the digestive tract, just to name a few of the changes observed.[9] So, an acute injury affects the body dramatically, but lesser stress also has a less obvious but cumulative long-term effect on the body and the metabolism.

Now, let's go to the bank: Imagine somebody wanted to borrow $5 from you. If you have $500 in the bank, a $5 loan isn't such a big deal. But what if you have only $10 in the bank? Suddenly, that $5 loan is pretty stressful. Let's look at stress a little differently—it's a natural part of life and something we can use rather than avoid at all costs. Instead of putting a value judgment on it, let's reframe it. But first, let's consider how your body perceives it.

Stress modifies the demands your body is under. For example, if you haven't eaten in 10 hours, or you're about to eat again after eating only thirty minutes before, or you haven't slept very well, or you're having a negative thought as you put food in your mouth (like "I shouldn't be eating this," or "I hope nobody sees me eating this"), every single one of these aspects of the environment determines what enzymes are secreted and what will happen as a consequence of that food in that particular environment—to your liver, gallbladder, pancreas, fat cells, and brain chemistry. Even the nerve cells in your teeny baby toe are affected in some way by the experience your whole body undergoes at every given moment.

Maybe your body is saying, "OMG, I'm starving and I haven't had lasagna in forever. This is going to make me feel so much better, and it was so kind of my neighbor to drop it off knowing I haven't felt well lately." That will create a very different internal environment and response to the food than if your body is saying, "I'm sad, I'm lonely, I'm depressed, I'm going to feel like shit forever. It doesn't matter what I put into my mouth because nothing is ever going to change." If you eat that exact same lasagna with these different feelings, the actual biochemical response to the food will be different, and will affect the way your metabolic pathways use or store fat and how they break down those lasagna nutrients to make them bio-available (or not).

How you eat can also affect the way your body handles stress. One dramatic way this happens is by changing the composition of your gut bacteria. What you eat can change the composition of this gut microflora within hours, and the composition of your gut bacteria can have a direct impact on your mood,[10] or even your food preferences,[11] making you crave sugar, or salt, or meat, or vegetables, or be relentlessly hungry, or not hungry at all.

Stress also leads to inflammation, and stress hormones like cortisol and adrenaline can cause inflammation in the tissues as a preemptive strike against injury; but in the absence of injury, the inflammation itself can become injurious. This can lead to problems absorbing and utilizing cholesterol—which can lead to heart disease—as well as higher blood sugar, which can lead to prediabetic conditions or even full-blown diabetes. Every one of these conditions is simply your body's attempt to deal with a changing environment—the potentially cataclysmic chain of events initially stemming from stress.

After all this chaos (which you may or may not be feeling in an obvious way as your body continues to whisper to you), your body shape begins to adapt, too, by storing fat for emergency use in all kinds of weird places—usually the places you least want fat to hang out. You'll also start feeling worse—lower on energy, with compromised performance, whether at work, in the bedroom, or at the gym. This can lead to poor food choices, saddle bags and cellulite and belly fat, more anxiety or depression, or even a chronic disease diagnosis. It leads to the decision to stay on the couch because you just don't feel good enough to go for a walk. It leads to poor self-esteem, to giving up, to fatalism. "I can't help it. It's in my genes." "It's the medication." "I am destined to be sick and fat."

None of this happens in a linear way—not even gene expression. Each system impacts every other symptom, so the interactions happen in three-dimensional feedback loops with no obvious beginning or end. And yet, you have control over all of it from the beginning, even if you don't know where it all began.

Adaptation is pretty amazing, and the cascade of metabolic adaptations happening inside your body in response to stress might be relatively straightforward or beyond your comprehension. For example, maybe you've been forgetting to drink enough water, and that has made you constipated. You might not realize that's why you are constipated, but your body has adapted to a dehydrated condition by holding on to everything containing fluid that it possibly can. The cascade might also be more complicated. Maybe you stopped eating grains and fruit because you heard this can help you lose weight. The lack of these foods in your diet may have caused you to be deficient in an enzyme that normally stimulates your thyroid, and now your thyroid has become inactive, causing your hair to fall out. You have no idea that a dietary decision has resulted in your hair loss because you didn't witness the biochemical changes that occurred as a result of the change in your internal environment.

To understand where this stress response starts—the stress response that is responsible for so much metabolic adaptation—let's take a closer look at your adrenal glands.

METABOLIC ADAPTATION AND YOUR ADRENAL GLANDS

It would be reductionist to think that there is just one isolated part of the body that is solely responsible for whole-body metabolic adaptation. Every part of the body is connected and interactive. However, much of the burden of metabolic adaptation sits on the shoulders of the adrenal glands.[12] The adrenals are an important part of your body's internal stress-management system. When your brain detects a stressful situation (positive or negative), it sends a message to your adrenals, which jump into action, sending chemical messages throughout the body and telling it what to do. These messages get sent along the line like a game of telephone, causing change after change after change in a vast network of metabolic adaptations.

It isn't only the adrenals sending out these messages, either; the adrenals work with all the other endocrine glands, especially the pituitary and the hypothalamus, which are interdependent in the way they orchestrate the stress response.[13] The adrenals do so much to regulate the body's stress response, however, that they have a major impact on how you adapt to a changing environment.

Your adrenals regulate glycogen levels, influencing blood sugar and insulin. They influence carbohydrate metabolism and cholesterol metabolism. They regulate blood pressure. They regulate hormone function, which affects nearly everything about your metabolism, including how and where you store fat. Through these pathways, the adrenals can influence a lot about how you feel and how healthy you are. The adrenals are responsible for the fluidity in your body's ability to adapt healthfully or not to changing circumstances, and this process must stay fluid for us to survive.

If your adrenals aren't nourished, they can interfere with your body's ability to physically interact with food—that is, digestion. If you aren't digesting your food, then you may not be providing the nutrients necessary for the production of serotonin (produced mostly in your gastrointestinal tract), and that can impact your mood in the form of mood disorders like depression, anxiety, and brain fog. This can cause further stress that can interfere with the immune system in a number of complex ways, which could send it into overdrive, leading to autoimmune disease.

If you learn how to read your body's signals, and what to eat in response to them, you can prevent most of the dysfunction, however. The questions you should be asking yourself and your body every day are: What are you adapting to? and How can I help? This is not a time to be reductionist. Is your body adapting to a high stress level? Too much or too little movement? Too much sugar or too much dietary fat? Where is the imbalance? Your body is always talking to you and trying to tell you where it is going off track. It is constantly trying to create some semblance of balance, or homeostasis, in the face of a constantly changing internal and external environment.

The best reason to pay closer attention to how your body is adapting to your current environment may not be about looking better. When your butt gets bigger or your waist gets wider or your arms get flabby, these are warning signs. To ignore them is to ignore the beginning stages of chronic disease.

I recently had a client who waited six months to see me because of my lengthy waiting list. When she finally got her turn, she marched into my office with a handful of medications, dropped them onto my desk, and said,

"That's it. I'm done. I took my last doses of this medication yesterday. Now it's your turn. My friend Caroline saw you, and she's off all her medications, and I want what she got."

"No, no, no," I told her. "That's not how it works. Caroline and I spent two and a half years getting her where she needs to be. If you were trying to drive from California to Florida and you took a wrong turn and ended up somewhere in the middle of Wyoming, you've got some miles still to cover. That doesn't mean you give up on the car and decide to walk to Florida."

So where are you now? Are you ready to start communicating with your body in a new way? Are you ready to start eating? Eating is nonnegotiable, but now we're going to make it strategic, really harnessing its power and potential.

There are things you cannot change, like the environmental chemicals in the air or water or your particular genetics. But you don't have to be a prisoner to a polluted environment or your genetic makeup. What you can change is your *internal environment*, and that can override the influences you can't change, including the way your body processes and eliminates that pollution, and the way your body expresses or doesn't express those genes. And you have an opportunity to change your internal environment *every single time you eat*. The foods you choose will specifically alter your metabolic pathways, helping to determine which are nourished and which are starved, what pathways get turned on and which get turned off, are blocked or are released. You have incredible power over your metabolism—just by changing the foods you eat. You can *eat to treat* in a way that's far more powerful than any medication. All you have to do is know which foods to choose. I'll show you.

You are adapting, right now, to the air you breathe, to the water you drink, to the things that happen in your life, to your most recent thoughts and feelings, to your stress, and especially to what you had at your last meal. Did you eat in order to adapt better, to optimize? Did you eat to survive, or to thrive? This is the time to think about yourself and to focus on yourself and recognize what your health issues are right now, because what's right for everybody else may not be what's right for you.

If you can't figure out how you got where you are, that's okay. We can find the way back to the main road by eating. Even if we don't know where you first took a wrong turn, we can get you going back in the direction you wanted to go: Toward the energy you used to have and the performance you used to enjoy; toward the body shape you desire; toward a stronger body, superior health, vigor; and toward achievement and optimism about your future. You need a food prescription, but the only way I can guide you properly is if you step up and pay attention to what your body is telling you. It's time to start listening. Your body has adapted to its environment in the best way it knows how. It's time to put some purpose on your plate.

If you want to change what your body is doing, you can do that with food. If you want to change how your metabolism is working, you can do that with food. If you want to repair specific metabolic pathways, you can do that with food. Whether your issue is large or small, whether it concerns you because you don't like the reflection in the mirror or because you really can't get out of bed, food will make the difference. I have a lifelong love affair with food, and I want you in on it. Food can save your life, even years before you ever realize it needs saving. Food is the answer, but it's going to take more than an apple a day.

CHAPTER 3

What Is Your Body Telling You?

If you do not change direction, you may end up where you are heading.
—Lao Tzu

Now it's time to get a little more intimate. (Insert Barry White music here?) What is your body trying to tell us? How can we best respond? What is going on with you and what are we going to do about it? How are you feeling? How are you doing? Are you dealing with crushing stress? Are you fatigued and exhausted? Do you feel sad more often than not? Are you quick to anger? Are you feeling foggy and uninspired? Are you bloated or gassy or constipated? Is your cholesterol high or your blood sugars out of control? Has a disease process already started in your body, and how can we turn it around? If we can figure out why the body is using dysfunction to survive, we can use food to repair the maladaptation and redirect the body to adapt in a way that results in the body and the health we desire. We can use food to shift from surviving to thriving.

Your body communicates with you all the time. Whether it's through brittle nails or hunger pains, bloating, insomnia, or emotional outbursts, it is communicating. Sometimes the style of communication is functional. For example, when your body gives you little signals that it's time to have a bowel movement, you can excuse yourself from a crowd and take care of business. Other times it's dysfunctional. For example, incontinence caused by a hormonal dysfunction can be a stressful way the body communicates that something is wrong. Every communication is important to me, whether your body is whispering, talking, or screaming. It matters and guides us to clues for repair.

When you take an interest in yourself, your body, and your symptoms, and how you feel and live, you get valuable information that will help you determine what to do. In fact, every single thing happening to you right now—from your sleep patterns to your energy level, your weight issues to your food preferences, your health philosophies to your bowel movements—all mean something. All of them. And I want us to explore them all. I want to help you to create an intimate dialogue with yourself and what your body is telling you, so we can determine what you need. Sometimes clients come in to my office and feel like it's all TMI (too much information) because, believe me, I ask a lot of questions. No. I say, let's connect the dots and get you a food prescription that can repair the dysfunctions. There is nothing your body is saying that's unimportant. You are too important.

I want to forge a connection between what you know about yourself and what science knows about your health disorder. I want to put the two of you together, and food's medicine is the connector. The right prescription can repair, restore, and rebalance your health.

Your metabolism is the engine and food is your fuel. How well is your engine running? Look at yourself. Feel how you feel. Listen to what your body is telling you. Don't look for answers or solutions yet. That can derail the internal conversation. Just be curious and listen.

The following list of questions resembles the intake form for my clinic. It is a self-assessment questionnaire that I give to my clients to help them start listening and pondering what is going on. Don't look for answers just yet—those will come later. This is the beginning of a conversation I want you to start having with your body. I don't proceed with my clients until they answer these questions. At the end of the list, you will find some blank spaces. I want you to add at least ten additional things to the list that you think your body would like to communicate to you. Remember, in my clinic, *anything* is up for discussion. It can be as seemingly minor as a muffin top or as major as heart disease:

SELF-ASSESSMENT QUESTIONNAIRE

Y = Yes; N = No; S = Sometimes

	Y	N	S	Details?
Is your energy low?				
Is your physical strength limited?				
Is your physical structure what you'd like?				
Do you have to drag yourself out of bed in the morning? Do you wake up feeling like you pulled an all-nighter?				
Do you long for a nap every afternoon?				
Are you having difficulty adapting to the stress you are under?				
Are you having trouble falling or staying asleep?				
Is your sex drive M.I.A.?				
Do you have trouble recovering after overindulging in food or alcohol? Are your hangovers (including the sugar-binge hangovers) harsher than they have ever been before?				
Are you unable to get the performance you need out of your body?				
Do you weigh more than you feel you should?				
Is your body depositing fatty tissue where it has never been before?				
Has your body changed into a shape you barely recognize?				
Do you have flabby upper arms?				
Do you have sagging skin on your face or neck?				
Do you have digestive issues like gas, bloating, constipation, heartburn, indigestion, or IBS?				
Are your periods irregular?				

Do you have hot flashes and/or brain fog?				
Do you have depression, anxiety, or mood swings?				
Do you have problems with focus, memory, concentration, or other cognition issues?				
Do you have an autoimmune disease, or a family history of autoimmune disorders?				
Do you have high cholesterol, elevated triglycerides, or low HDL?				
Do you have high blood pressure?				
Do you have systemic inflammation?				
Do you have high blood sugar, are you insulin resistant, or do you have full-blown diabetes?				
Have you been diagnosed with a disease or disorder?				

More issues you have noticed:	Details?
1.	
2.	
3.	
4.	
5.	
6.	
7.	
8.	
9.	
10.	
11.	
12.	
13.	

These responses indicate evidence of conversations your body is having with you. Something is off with your metabolism, and that means your body is metabolically adapting to an environment that isn't right for it. Maybe your body is whispering, talking, or even screaming for your attention. Your body has acted heroically by adapting, and we can and should be thankful for that. When we listen and stop looking at these things as complaints, but instead see them as requests for repair, then we can design a plan that meets your unique metabolic needs. My goal here is to give you the tools to say, "I hear you and I am ready to feed your metabolic needs."

LOST IN TRANSLATION: WHEN YOU AREN'T LISTENING OR NOT QUITE GETTING THE MESSAGE

Long before you manifest disease, your body has been talking to you. It has been talking to you for years. It has been talking to you since birth. Every time your environment changes, your body adapts and lets you know. It adapts to the foods you eat, the air you breathe, the toxins you are exposed to, the nutrients you give it, the things you do, and the thoughts you think. If your body didn't have this valuable skill, you would be in big trouble every time you ate a doughnut, or went outside on a cold winter day, or had to run away from a threat, or inhaled pollution.

When you eat sugar, for example, your body metabolically adapts to the changing internal environment by releasing insulin to help move the sugar into the right places—to your brain or your muscles, or your liver or your fat cells. If you go outside on a very cold day, your body knows to constrict your blood vessels to conserve heat. If you are suddenly under threat, your body sends fuel to your muscles so you can move faster and it dilates your pupils for better vision. When you inhale polluted air, your body's natural detoxification system takes over and shuttles those toxins safely back out of the body or stores them where they can't hurt you.

One of the most basic examples of metabolic adaptation is what happens when you eat: Your body responds by producing a particular set of enzymes to digest the food you chose to eat. Even before you taste that food, as you smell it or prepare it, your body picks up signals: *What are we eating today? What do we need to do to get ready for that food?* This is a type of metabolic adaptation. If your body senses incoming sugar, or meat, or bread, or fat, ei-

Many of my clients tell me they can't lose weight or avoid chronic illnesses because it is in their genes. Focusing on genetics can be a reductionist approach. We all have our genetic tendencies, but they are far from destiny. That simplistic belief about genetics is as wrong as when people believed the earth was flat. Loosen the grip on that story! Science is showing us that gene expression is determined metabolically.

Research has demonstrated that many genes can be turned on or off based on environment, and that includes lifestyle choices like food, stress, and exposure to toxins and viruses. To use one example, you could have a genetic propensity for heart disease, but if you tweak your environment in a way that never turns on those genes, you could avoid heart disease. (Research is now showing that even if a gene has been turned on, it can be turned off again.) If you come from a family with weight issues or cholesterol issues or depression issues, those are symptoms that something is not being supported in those individuals, not that something is unalterable about the family line. If you really look at the science, you will learn that genetics is mutable.

You have the ability to adapt. It is in your very DNA. More specifically, the food you eat determines which metabolic pathway you go down on any given day. Food can lead a gene to express itself, whether good or bad. Food can lead a gene to stay dormant—also whether good or bad. The science of this phenomenon is called *epigenetics*.

The notion that genes guide destiny is, in fact, a special kind of danger in medicine because it makes clients apathetic about invoking change. I have thirty-five-year-old men coming in to my clinic who are on cholesterol medication, who tell me stories of their fathers having died of heart attacks at age fifty-four. Their doctors told them they were genetically predisposed to have elevated cholesterol, and that statin drugs are their only savior. I can't tell you how many times I have used food with those clients to get them off statins. Food can be that powerful.

ther through smell or taste, or even the thought of those foods you know you are about to eat, it will set a chemical chain reaction in motion so you can best digest what's coming in and take the best possible advantage of those nutrients. These are all metabolic adaptations that make sense and have an obviously positive result.

Metabolic adaptation can also result in things you don't like, but this isn't your body's fault. Your body is just keeping you alive. If your hair is falling out, or your skin quality is poor, or you have no energy, or you have developed back fat or a belly, or if you are depressed or are told you are prediabetic, or have high blood pressure, or high cholesterol, or an autoimmune disease, you might feel that your body has betrayed you. However, these are the *exact things that are saving your life.* When your body doesn't have the nutrients to support full-body maintenance, it knows to sacrifice the least important things first. It knows that the appearance of your hair and skin is less important than the functioning of your heart and liver, so it sends its limited resources where they are most needed. Here are some other examples:

- If your body doesn't have the resources to fortify deep reparative sleep, it knows it must conserve energy, so it gives you less energy for things like exercise.

- If you aren't providing the right nutrients to properly absorb sugar or balance the salt in your blood, or if your biochemistry isn't supporting cholesterol metabolism, your body goes into crisis mode. You get diabetes, or high blood pressure, or high cholesterol because your body is working in the best way it knows how to manage those imbalances without killing you immediately.

- If your toxic overload is too much for your body to handle, it will fill your fat cells with those toxins to protect you, or it might even develop an overactive immune response to try to fight off invaders, and that can turn into an autoimmune disease. These toxins can build up over time to become chronic exposures, or they can be episodic, like a one-time heavy chemical exposure or an infection.

It's not your body's fault if it doesn't get everything it needs to produce glowing health. Sometimes, the low energy, fat accumulation, even the chronic disease is your body's only option. You have diabetes so you won't die. Blood sugar surges can kill you in a very short time, so your body manages roller-coaster blood sugar levels by adapting in a way that might kill you eventually, but won't kill you *right now.* You have heart disease because your body is protecting you. Your body is managing the tears and damage to your arterial lining by patching them with plaque and attempting to calm the inflammation. You may die from heart disease eventually, but it won't kill you as fast as an arterial rupture or a blood infection. You have an autoimmune disorder because that is the best way your body can deal with the stress of managing foreign substances in places they aren't supposed to be. Yes, you can eventually die from autoimmune disease, but it won't kill you as fast as a foreign body that could kill you immediately.

Some people say the body gets confused, mistaking (for example) its own tissue for an invader, but I don't believe the body gets confused. Autoimmunity, heart disease, and diabetes all happen as metabolic adaptations in the body that begin much sooner than when you need insulin shots or a triple bypass or when your body starts attacking your own thyroid or joints or neural tissue. These are metabolic adaptations designed for survival. Your body is smart. Never forget that. So let's start listening. This is important, and it can make a big difference in how well you thrive.

YOUR BODY'S MESSAGES

Here are some of the messages you might be able to hear right now.

WHEN YOUR BODY IS WHISPERING

At first, your body whispers. It sends you subtle messages that all is not working right, that it is not getting everything it needs (like certain nutrients), or that it is getting too much of something it doesn't need. This is when you will experience subtle signs of dysfunction, like problems with digestion or elimination (such as constipation) and a downshift in energy. When your body is whispering, you may notice that all is not going as well as it could, but you might not think to seek out medical care. Metabolic adaptations that are but whispers are often things people just think they are supposed to deal with—fatigue, sleep issues, weight gain, monthly irritability or weepiness, or low energy. At worst, these may be a footnote at a doctor's visit: "By the way, doctor, I've been really tired," or "I'm not sure why I gained fifteen pounds this year." This is also what I call the "of course" stage: "Of course, you're tired! You work hard!" "Of course, you've gained weight. You just turned forty." "Of course, your skin is sagging. You've had too much sun exposure." "Of course, you have hot flashes—it's perimenopause." "Of course, you are irritable or weepy. It's just PMS. It happens to everyone."

The problem is that it doesn't happen to everyone, and none of these "whispers" is something that you have to accept or suffer with in silence. They are messages that something is going wrong, and they are sent to you because you are the one who can set things right . . . if you listen.

Although metabolism is complex and can whisper to you in many ways, these are the two most common situations I see when the body first starts to indicate a problem:

- *IBS, Indigestion, and Other GI Dysfunction.* When inflammation and an imbalanced gut flora population begin to interfere with the smooth operation of your digestive tract and the assimilation of nutrients from food, the result is often IBS (irritable bowel syndrome) and/or indigestion. This manifests in symptoms like gas, bloating, constipation, diarrhea, acid reflux, and heartburn. Large particles of food are likely making their way too far down the GI tract because they aren't being broken down properly, and this creates a reaction to the food as if it were foreign matter. The body has been unable to access the micronutrients from this undigested food, inhibiting the functionality of other metabolic pathways. Finally, the receptor sites for proper immune function and brain chemistry modulation become compromised, setting the stage for depression and autoimmune disorders.

  GI dysfunction is often at the root of many other disorders because if you can't digest the nutrients in your food, you can disrupt many metabolic pathways that control the regulation of hormones, blood sugar and insulin, and lipid metabolism. Our goal here is to get the digestive system moving again and also to replenish the gut bacteria that promote health rather than digestive upset. This way, your IBS and indigestion symptoms cannot just disappear for now but can be resolved permanently—and you can start using all the nutrients you need from the foods you eat.

- *Fatigue, Low Energy, and Exhaustion.* When you experience fatigue, low energy, and/or exhaustion, there are several reasons this can happen. One reason is that the body isn't accessing the available nutrients because of either reduced uptake (ability to take and use nutrients) or a reduced ability to convert nutrients to energy in the cell. Another reason is that the end products of cell metabolism aren't being delivered as energy. In other words, things can break down all along the metabolic pathways for energy metabolism, and when this happens, you start to feel different. You get tired more easily. Exercise seems more difficult. Your sex drive fades. You might also notice thinner, dryer hair, skin, and nails because your body needs energy to make these, and it will pull energy from the functions it determines are less important to your survival. Your athletic performance may also decline—if you aren't making enough energy, you aren't going to be able to run that 5K like you can when you are making sufficient amounts. In other words, your body is adapting to fewer resources by conserving energy in any way it can. That means you have less energy for all the things you want to do, from sex, to your workout, to just getting through the day without falling asleep. We need to feed the four pathways of energy metabolism in the body (I'll explain these in Chapter 6, on energy) so you have as much energy as you need.

Early metabolic adaptations may seem harmless or more relevant to convenience (you can get more done with more energy) or vanity (you will look better if you don't have that bloated belly) than health, but when allowed to proceed unchecked or uncontrolled, they can eventually result in dysfunction of your organ systems. This leaves them to no longer properly metabolize cholesterol, regulate blood pressure, balance hormones, or juggle the constant fluctuations in blood sugar and insulin. When that happens, you won't just be unhappy with how you feel or the reflection in the mirror. You will be ill. So let's get this under control right now.

WHEN YOUR BODY IS TALKING

If you don't listen, then your body is going to have to raise its voice. It won't have to get too loud yet, but it will start talking to you in ways you might be more likely to hear: hormonal imbalances that result in uncomfortable symptoms like PMS or brain fog, hot flashes, low libido, sleep disruption, and other symptoms of perimenopause (or for guys, low testosterone) and its accompanying symptoms, like low sex drive and low energy. You might develop skin rashes, food or environmental allergies, dark circles under your eyes, mood changes like depression or anxiety, or elevated blood cholesterol, triglycerides, or inflammation levels. When your body is talking, your doctor may also suggest medication, especially if your symptoms are interfering with your life. Your doctor isn't necessarily *worried* at this point about common hormonal symptoms, mood changes, or slightly elevated lipid labs; in fact, the doctor may be glad he or she can offer you a simple solution: hormone replacement (such as birth control) perhaps, or maybe an antidepressant or a statin medication. If the issue doesn't seem severe, it may be a "no big deal—just take this drug to feel more comfortable" type of situation. In our current medical climate, until you manifest actual, diagnosable disease, you are "fine."

The problem is, once you start muffling the body's voice with medication, you won't be able to hear its messages anymore. You'll be putting a gag on your body's voice, which practically guarantees you won't do anything to change your course, and that can drive you further into dysfunction and closer to disease.

When the body starts to speak up for itself, it can happen in many ways, but these are the three metabolic adaptations I often see in my clients when the body's environment has changed and the body is metabolically adapting in a more insistent way:

- *PMS, Perimenopause, Menopause, and "Manopause."* When your hormones get out of balance, it is a sign that your body is talking more loudly. This means the glands that create and regulate hormonal release and absorption aren't sufficiently nourished, and they are losing function. This is a serious issue because hormones influence almost every process in your body. They are major metabolic players. At the very beginning, when they just start to shift, you will notice smaller changes, like worsening PMS, perimenopause, and what I call "manopause," which is a blanket term for the hormonal imbalances (such as low testosterone) that men frequently experience. In addition, your fat cells may have begun to create compensatory hormones from cholesterol, which can interfere with your hormonal balance, as well as lipid balance. Another downstream effect is that the body's ability to manufacture vitamin D often becomes compromised. To treat hormonal imbalance with food, we want to nourish the endocrine glands that produce hormones, and also clear out or wash the hormone receptors so they can actually use the hormones our bodies produce.

- *Impaired Cholesterol Metabolism.* Cholesterol gets a bad rap, but it is actually an extremely valuable and beneficial substance your body, and particularly your brain, requires. If you lose the ability to metabolize it efficiently due to insufficient support of the metabolic pathways for cholesterol metabolism—and most particularly, insufficient nourishment of the liver that metabolizes cholesterol—this liquid gold can begin to collect in your blood (having nowhere else to go). This can result in "high cholesterol," which your doctor will tell you is a serious risk factor for heart disease. But the problem isn't that you ate cholesterol. The problem is that you aren't metabolizing cholesterol. Instead of being metabolized into hormones that stimulate mood, energy, sex hormone production, blood sugar stabilization, immune function, blood pressure regulation, and body structure development and repair, cholesterol begins to hang out in the blood—especially the "bad" kind (LDL) most associated with an increased risk of heart disease. The "good" cholesterol (HDL) most associated with a decreased risk in heart disease begins to decline. This creates inflammation, which inhibits sex hormone uptake and increases fat cell accumulation. You may also notice a decrease in memory and cognition. Production of bile salts becomes compromised, lowering the body's ability to break down fats and cholesterol, creating a deficiency in hormones, vitamin D, and impacting brain chemistry. This signals the body to slow cholesterol metabolism down even further. What we want to do for the body in this situation is to nourish the gallbladder to produce bile salts and clear out the pathways for cholesterol metabolism so your body can use that liquid gold!

- *Mood Changes and Cognitive Challenges.* When you experience troublesome mood changes like depression or anxiety, or cognitive difficulties like brain fog, attention problems, or hyperactivity, you can be sure there is a breakdown in your body's ability to convert bioactive substances and transport hormones to the correct receptor sites in your central nervous system. In the case of a biochemical cause, much of this happens in the GI tract, where most of your serotonin is produced and where you have a concentration of neurological cells that communicate with the brain, so the right food is particularly useful in correcting the imbalance. Anxiety and depression often go hand in hand and sometimes overlap because when we stop making and transporting, and absorbing and converting, bioactive neurotransmitters like serotonin and dopamine, the body starts trying to balance itself out. Remember, the body's number one job is to survive in its current environment. Serotonin may be the optimal neurotransmitter, contributing to waking and mood and good cognitive reasoning skills, and even the ability to feel joy. But if serotonin is depleted because of imbalance in the gut biome, or because of nutrient deficiencies or a genetic predisposition, the body will produce adrenal hormones to keep the mechanisms of the brain working, albeit in a dysfunctional way. The body often does this by secreting things like epinephrine, norepinephrine, and dopamine, which can lead to mood and cognition disruption. Think about those moments when you are really hungry but don't have anything healthy to eat in the fridge. You feel you have to eat, but your only choice is junk food because that's all you have. This is your brain, surviving without sufficient serotonin or with blocked neurotransmitter receptor sites, or whatever the particular dysfunction may be. It gets by on the biochemicals it can find and use. Life marches on and you do what you can, and so does your body. Take a chemical like cortisol, the so-called stress hormone. Cortisol can be a wonderful thing. It makes you feel good. It makes you happy. It wakes you up. It dilates your blood vessels and increases blood flow to the brain and heart. It is elevated when you wake up in the morning, and it should be low when you go to bed. It helps to contribute to the circadian rhythm in a way that keeps you balanced and feeling like yourself. When all is working properly you have optimal mood and health.

But if, to continue the example, the sun goes down and your body hasn't completed all its work for the day (of repair, building, expending energy), the body can excrete crisis hormones: *I'm not ready for bed yet!* This is why people often experience anxiety in the late afternoon, or have heart palpitations or feelings of anxiety at bed time. The body may be saying, "Oh no. I'm going into a dormant state and I still have toxicity I won't be able to handle! I don't know what to do with it except store it away as fat, or it might hurt me." Then we wake up feeling fatigued and lethargic.

When the receptor sites for neurotransmitters are blocked, we can get foggy, depressed, confused, or distracted. There is a time to be sleepy and lack motivation, but it is not the morning—it should be at bedtime! There is time to have a surge of energy, even "worry hormones," but it is not at bedtime. It should be at the peak of your daytime activity. Fix the hormones, restore the circadian rhythm through regular habits and good sleep hygiene, and repair the mechanisms for hormone metabolism, and you will notice that your moods begin to stabilize and your cognitive abilities improve.

WHEN YOUR BODY IS SCREAMING

Finally, when your body is completely frustrated with you, it will begin screaming. The screams are disease states—conditions you might be diagnosed with because you've not listened before. I'm talking about autoimmune diseases like multiple sclerosis and rheumatoid arthritis and lupus, and pre-diabetic states like metabolic syndrome that eventually are likely to lead to full-blown diabetes. This is when surgery and hospitalization are not uncommon. Diabetics get ulcers and sometimes need to have toes removed. People can be hospitalized for a wide variety of health emergencies that can result from autoimmune diseases. Medications like insulin shots and immunosuppressive drugs come into play, and these have even more severe side effects than the earlier meds. In our current medical climate, the louder the body's voice, the stronger the drug. How about instead saying, "Hey, wait a minute, what's wrong? Why are you yelling at me?"

This is also the stage when you become a "sick person." This is the stage when your illness begins to define you. It becomes your identity. You are a diabetic. You are the doctor's "MS patient" or "lupus patient." You have heart disease. You are labeled, and it can be very difficult for you (and your poor body) to get out from under that label, not just in terms of what the medical community calls you but also in terms of what you call yourself and how you feel about who you are and the daily fear that comes with it.

The problem is, you are not "a diabetic" or "the MS patient." You are not a disease. You are *you*. You are a person, and this is just something that is happening to you, temporarily, in this stage of your life. The body is constantly in flux. There are a million diagnoses, but they are only labels. Giving somebody a diagnosis has never cured anything. What's important is the message behind the diagnosis. Your body is in a more desperate state than when it was just whispering to you, but it is still asking you for things. It is still trying to tell you what it needs. And there is still time to listen. As long as you're alive, it's never too late to listen.

- *Autoimmune Issues.* There are many different autoimmune conditions, from multiple sclerosis to lupus, celiac disease to Hashimoto's thyroiditis, to rheumatoid arthritis (and many more), but they all have one thing in common: The immune system has overreacted and turned on itself, attacking healthy tissue in the body with "friendly fire" as it tries to fight off sometimes mild, latent infections or chronic toxicity loads. This disrupts the metabolic pathways that regulate hormones and the neurotransmitters that affect the skin and sensory organs, creating a wide range of symptoms and multisensory reactions in the body. You could suffer from rashes or joint pain, loss of mobility or blood sugar modulation, carbohydrate resistance, or spleen, bone marrow, and mineral distribution that has become imbalanced. This continues to send mixed messages to the immune system. Fight-or-flight hormones from the adrenal glands may also become imbalanced, creating a new normal where your body adapts to, or learns to live with, this chronic dysfunction. Leaky gut may also be involved: inflammation and gut lining damage can result in protein particles escaping into the bloodstream and triggering the immune system. Your body is metabolically adapting to the presence of immune threats, and it believes these threats are extreme and imminent. Repairing digestion is crucial in treating autoimmunity with food, and so is the careful elimination of any reactive food substances that could be contributing to gut inflammation and immune system reactivity as the body relearns how to exercise its immune system appropriately. It might appear as if the body thinks nothing of destroying its own cells. But listen carefully: Your body is doing all this to survive.

- *Prediabetes, Metabolic Syndrome, and Type 2 Diabetes.* Prediabetes, prediabetic conditions like metabolic syndrome, and full-blown type 2 diabetes are notorious conditions involving blood sugar and insulin. They are commonly believed to be caused by eating too much sugar. However, you don't get diabetes from eating sugar. You get diabetes when your body loses the ability to metabolize sugar. When you don't use sugar for energy, sugar stays in your bloodstream. When you have too much sugar in your bloodstream, your pancreas responds by secreting more insulin. This triggers the adrenals to produce stress and crisis hormones, which in turn down-regulate energy formation. To try to create more energy, the body begins to access extra sugars from the smooth muscle and from the heart and liver, adding additional stress to the process of cholesterol metabolism, mood modulation, and infection defense. (Notice how all the health issues in this book are coming together and contributing their dysfunctional pathways to this particular process.) All this can result in a prediabetic condition, and eventually results in diabetes, a serious and sometimes fatal condition that requires careful medical management. The trick here isn't to eliminate all natural sugars and carbs, but to bolster the systems that manage sugar metabolism in order to keep the blood sugar and insulin steady and functional.

HEALING FROM THE TOP DOWN

Although these metabolic adaptations don't necessarily occur in this order in everyone, there is a traditional healing theory (homotoxicology, the study of how the body processes toxins and nutrition) that says the body tends to heal from the top down, from the inside out, and from the newest symptom to the oldest symptom. Also, traditional healers say it typically takes about a month of food therapy for every year that the imbalance has been in place. I find this to be true in my practice. For example, I have a client who has dealt with chronic constipation for his entire life—about forty years. Even though this is his body "whispering," it was a long-term insistent whisper that needed more time—a good forty months—to become quiet as the chronic constipation was gently reversed. We had gotten the bowels moving fairly easily using food, but it took much longer to repair the underlying dysfunction in the gastrointestinal tract that triggered the constipation.

It is a slow, but sure process. By contrast, someone who is just starting to notice an energy downshift over the past few weeks can correct this underlying issue much more quickly with food therapy. If you've had diabetes for six years, you may feel better in a week with a food prescription, but it will take somewhere around six months to start reversing the actual diabetic condition using food.

When the body is whispering, it may be able to repair itself quickly, if you listen. Maybe your body has been whispering to you with fatigue and low energy, but it has never felt the need to scream. Or maybe you just didn't have the energy to scream—maybe your whisper is really a whimper. It can be easy to misinterpret the body's intent by underestimating the seriousness or destructive potential of its messages, especially the quieter ones. Because yes, often times, the squeaky wheel is the one that gets greased.

When the body is talking, it might also be something that can be resolved quickly. A new manifestation of high cholesterol or anxiety might be relatively quickly corrected with food therapy. Yet debilitating hormonal issues or persistently high lipid values or clinical depression can be pretty serious. Just because the body is talking and not screaming with a life-threatening diagnosis (by modern medical standards), that doesn't mean you shouldn't get right on the issue.

When the body is screaming, it may take longer to effect a repair because, in most cases, the body didn't just start screaming out of nowhere. There has probably been a long chain of dysfunction and repeated attempts at communication that weren't addressed. Still, food therapy can directly and effectively address the issue.

In our society, we think that if you scream something, it must be a big deal—and it often is. Yet many whispers in our world are the only warning signs that something is going wrong. Some warnings are quieter, less obvious, or less understood. For example, you will see in Chapter 5 that messages like gastrointestinal upset (things like IBS and indigestion) and also low energy, fatigue, and exhaustion, are "whispers." That's because we don't necessarily have a way to define low energy or digestive dysfunction the way we do a more recognized disease state, such as diabetes or multiple sclerosis. When you are getting whispers from your body, it may be a bit more difficult to convince a doctor that you need support.

When your body starts talking, intervention (and I am specifically talking about food intervention here) is generally more accepted. Your doctor may agree that you can try food therapy to help your PMS symptoms or lower your cholesterol or alleviate your depression. When your body is screaming, though, the medical community is quick to prescribe pharmaceuticals. If you have a serious case of diabetes, you may be prescribed insulin and/or a drug like metformin. If you have an autoimmune disease, your doctor may urge you to go on immunosuppressant drug therapy. From my point of view, food can be either a significant complement to those drug therapies or a replacement for them.

Every single one of the conditions in this book has a range of severity. Remember in Chapter 2, when I told you about the standard rubric for chronic disease? Chronic disease is multifaceted. It can whisper, talk, or scream. And it progresses. Whispers can get louder. Talking can turn into a scream. And even a whisper, if it goes on and on for years, can do some serious damage. Just because your body is whispering, that doesn't mean you should ignore it until it gets louder. Remain curious about your unique body's health journey. When you almost drive off the side of the road because you have a flat tire, you need to address that tire. Maybe you ran over a nail and the other tires are perfectly fine. But maybe the other tires are bald and cracked, and just because they also didn't scream and almost kill you, that doesn't mean you should ignore them until they do.

The good news is that metabolic adaptation works in multiple directions. No matter how far in the wrong direction you have traveled, you can always turn and head back toward a better way. And never forget that while symptom relief is important, the real point of food therapy is to repair the tissues in ways that the metabolic pathways can reroute themselves, and readapt to the new, nutrient-rich environment. The amazing thing about food therapy is that this repair is even possible.

What I want to do for you is help you read your body's messages and then give you *the one best thing to fix* your situation. Fix one metabolic pathway that is out of order, and you can create a cascade of functioning that can repair all the processes downstream. This is the way to talk back to your body—to say, "Hey, I hear you and I've got this." Every time the internal environment changes (which is constantly), it is like reaching a fork in the road. Will you go to the left or will you go to the right? Your metabolism has to decide, and it decides based on the resources it has onboard. There are millions of metabolic forks in the road that we face every day, and our bodies are constantly adapting by choosing left or right, or by slowing down, or stopping, or accelerating, or doing a U-turn. If you get a flat tire, or your tire is leaking air, you have a decision to make: Do you slow down? Do you stop and change the tire? Or do you ignore it and barrel down the interstate at top speed, destroying your wheels? If you are about to run out of fuel, do you hot-rod around the neighborhood? Do you stop for groceries before dealing with the problem? Or do you go straight to the gas station for a fill-up?

If you chose the left road when you should have chosen the right, I hear you. I've been through it. The choices you make can be life-altering, life-affirming, even potentially life-ending; your body can only work with what you give it. So let's begin by laying a healthy foundation for true metabolic repair.

CHAPTER 4

Foundational Foods: Laying the Groundwork for True Repair

Whether you believe you can do a thing or not, you are right.
    —Henry Ford

Now it's time to take this paradigm shift we've been talking about and apply it to your life. I'm going to take you through everything I would say and do if you were sitting in my office. First, we are going to make sure you have completed the Self-Assessment Questionnaire in Chapter 3. Then we're going to make sure you understand your prescription. After that, we are going to assemble your Health Dream Team. Next, I'll show you how to read and make your own meal map, explain how to fit movement into your life in an appropriate way, and finally, help you select what foods to eat based on the Foundational Foods List. By the end of this chapter, you will be fully prepared to begin a specific nutritional prescription for the health challenge you want to tackle first.

UNDERSTANDING YOUR BIG PICTURE

In the spirit of remaining curious, you may feel as if you picked up this book with an idea of where you were going to start. You know what problem you have or what issue you want to resolve. But this book is as much about self-exploration as it is about me or your doctor, or anybody else's dictating what's right for you. This book conveys a process that I take my clients through.

I can't tell you how many times, based on those intake forms, I have a good idea of what these new clients' nutrition plans will be. But after we've spent time being curious about what's going on in their bodies, they often walk out the door with something different from those first ideas. For example, maybe you know you want to deal with your mood issues, but through exploration, you discover that those mood issues are really symptoms of something else, like a hormone imbalance or an inability to properly metabolize cholesterol (which creates the hormones responsible for mood modulation), or maybe even that your inability to concentrate was really a symptom of an autoimmune condition.

I have provided a longer questionnaire in Chapter 12—Your Whole-Body Diagnosis Quiz—to enable further exploration, but before you tackle it, read the rest of this book. You may think you don't have a specific health issue, but learning about it may change your mind. Or, you may be sure you have one particular issue, but reading the chapters that follow may help you see that it is really a metabolic side effect of something else. All these issues are intertwined, because all parts of your body work together. The more you know about yourself, the better you can feed yourself. Knowledge is at the crux of not only action but also prevention.

There is a piece of you in every chapter of this book, and maybe that piece is shining bright and doing great—but maybe it's in a state of metabolic dysfunction. I like to say, "All of it is in every bit of it," meaning every dysfunction, no matter how small, is representative of the state of your entire body. Small-scale problems are reflected in whole-body health. See how you resonate with what's in these chapters—not just the individual, stand-alone symptoms but also the symptom profiles of each issue discussed in these next seven chapters. Explore them and then—and only then—decide where you should start.

Preferably, return to the Self-Assessment Questionnaire in Chapter 3 and take a look at it. (If you haven't already done so, fill it in now.) You would not be admitted to my office until you filled out this questionnaire, after which we would go through it together. So, look at your list of what is bothering you and what you want to accomplish. Do you already have an idea of where you want to start? What bothers you the most? Then go back and look at your Health

Wish List from Chapter 1. Think about everything you want for yourself, and believe that you can make those things happen. I want you to begin with a realistic picture of what is going on with you right now, but I also want you to know that the sky is the limit in terms of what we can accomplish together.

GUIDELINES FOR THE GENERAL RX

The next thing we would do if you were in my office is go over your general food prescription: What you will establish as a baseline before we tailor it to address the specific condition or issue you wish to repair. And just as you would get a prescription from a doctor with specific directions for when and how to take your medicine, I will give you instructions for when and how to take your specific nutritional prescription. As you work through the individual chapters, you will see more issue-specific advice, but the guidelines in this chapter apply to any and all issues and all prescriptions, so take note! Here are the seven principles necessary for your food prescription to work as it is intended:

1. YOU WILL BEGIN THE DAY WITH FOOD.

I want you to eat within thirty minutes of waking—always, every day, even if it is just a snack. I can already hear the excuses: "I'm not hungry when I first wake up," "Nothing sounds good to me first thing in the morning," and so on. I understand, and to those complaints I will only say: None of that matters if you really want to heal.

There is a natural physiological process that happens when you wake up in the morning. Your heart rate, blood pressure, and respiration rate all begin to rise. Your temperature goes up, too. Your platelets tend to coagulate, and your brain wave patterns change as you awaken, shifting from long, slow waves to shallower, faster waves.

There is also a complex excretion and suppression of many different hormones and neurotransmitters that help your body transition from the sleeping state to waking. All these changes have specific micronutrient needs, and if you aren't meeting their needs, those systems might not work as well as they should. Whenever your body is in a state of transition (the transition from waking to sleeping being one of the most crucial), eating can guide your metabolism in the right direction. These morning micronutrients can put your train on the right track, headed toward your desired destination.

Indeed, your entire day is full of potential opportunities for changing the structure of your body and the flavor of your mood. As your life changes, your nutrient needs change, too. Will you degrade your tissues—or build them? Will you support the mood you want—or foil it? Will you remodel muscle—or add fat?

One good example of how this works is in regard to insulin. The way insulin works in the first half of the day is different from the way it works in the second half. Insulin output tends to decline after 2:00 p.m. in the average body, on an average day, under average demands. Insulin is a storage hormone that determines whether the sugar you eat (whether in the form of a piece of bread, a piece of fruit, or a candy bar) will be taken into the cell to be burned for fuel or to be stored as fat. This is why I ask you to eat differently in the morning than in the evening. How you feed yourself in the first half of the day versus the second half has everything to do with whether you are supporting or fighting your body's natural cycle of insulin output.

Another example is cortisol, the so-called stress hormone. Cortisol is an important hormone that you need. It ensures that your heart keeps beating when you arise from your bed in the morning. You need that cortisol in the morning, but if cortisol is elevated in the afternoon, it can lead to insulin resistance and your body will be much more likely to turn that sugar you eat directly into belly fat. This happens because, as the day goes on, the signals from the neurotransmitters that regulate cravings are blocked by the increased insulin output that isn't supposed to be there. These neurotransmitters are supposed to signal when you are full, but if the receptors are blocked, you will be hungry. This can lead to excessive eating in the evening, which inhibits deep sleep, which in turn creates more cortisol because a sleep-deprived body is a stressed-out body.

Eating is always the path to better health. The metabolism is complex, but eating within thirty minutes of waking up gives you the best chance to set things right for the rest of the day.

Some people are in the habit of skipping breakfast. Maybe that habit started in an attempt to cut calories; maybe they just aren't hungry in the morning. Lately, there have been some prominent folks out there saying that you really should skip breakfast, and that this can actually be good for you. The suggestion horrifies me. Skip breakfast? Try not giving your dog its breakfast, and you could get turned in to the Humane Society. Try doing that to your horse, and then deal with the colic.

I understand that you have energy stores. You have a reserve of fuel on your rear end and sugar in your liver, so you might not collapse if you don't eat before noon, but how are you supposed to build and repair? You don't remodel your bones or muscles with sugar, and you don't store micronutrients anywhere in your body, with a very few exceptions. You could pull some calcium and other minerals from your muscles, including your heart muscle, which your body could cannibalize if necessary—cardiovascular sandwich, anyone? You store some iodine in your thyroid and some trace minerals in your bones, which your body could snack on in an emergency. Other than that, if you are undertaking the full-time job of living, you have to get your micronutrients from somewhere, and eating within thirty minutes of waking is the easiest, healthiest, and most pleasurable way to do that.

Some might argue that not eating in the morning gives the GI tract a break from being insulted by food, but I say: How about we just stop being so insulting? How about stopping the eating of foods that insult the GI tract, and start eating foods that nurture and repair it? Skipping breakfast is like deciding to be a shut-in because somebody wasn't nice to you. How about surrounding yourself with nice people instead?

I am always game for a new concept. I don't think I have all the answers, all the time. But when a suggestion like skipping breakfast comes along like this, I just want to say, "Hey, walk me through this and show me how it works." There are certain micronutrient-absorption processes and electrolyte-balancing processes that *cannot happen* until chewing and swallowing happen. We know this for a fact. It simply doesn't happen any other way. Even if you eat lunch like an angel, your body has already down-regulated to adapt to what you didn't do when you woke up. Grandma wasn't wrong. Her cookies *are* the best, and breakfast is the most important meal of the day.

"Gee, Haylie, why don't you tell us how you really feel?" Well, now you know. I just don't get it. I get fasting for religious or spiritual reasons—that's called a higher purpose. Dieting is not a higher purpose, but health is—and skipping breakfast is definitely not the path to that goal!

2. YOU WILL ALWAYS EAT THREE MEALS AND TWO TO THREE SNACKS EVERY DAY.

If you were taking a medication to regulate your cholesterol or your blood sugar, would you tell your doctor that you didn't feel like taking it? This is how I feel about food. You have to eat, and you have to eat regularly. You may not skip a single dose. That means three meals and two to three snacks (depending on your issues) every day.

Chronic dieters often have a problem with this. They think that if they skip meals, they will lose more weight. Yet exactly the opposite is true. If a doctor gave you medicine and you didn't know how it worked or you didn't see results right away, would you tell your doctor you weren't going to take it anymore? This is just like saying, "I'm going to do what Haylie says and resolve my diabetes/hypertension/cholesterol/obesity by eating"—and then choosing not to eat. Forget that. On my watch, you are eating three meals and two snacks every day. Every time you eat, you have the opportunity to change your body in positive ways. Don't miss an opportunity!

Here is your basic template:

Breakfast	Snack	Lunch	Snack	Dinner	Snack
					(Optional if you are still up 4 hours after finishing dinner, or if indicated for your prescription.)

How you time all this depends on when you sleep. As long as you start within thirty minutes of waking each day and eat every three to four hours while you're awake, you will be fueling your metabolism.

3. YOU WILL ALWAYS HAVE A SNACK BEFORE YOU EXERCISE.

I like to say "Don't fast before you go fast" because this is very important. Although some people say they like to exercise on an empty stomach, and this is even trendy, the simple fact is that micronutrients fuel exercise and movement, and if you don't provide the fuel, your body will make bio-adaptations that are not conducive to repairing broken metabolic pathways. Your body needs fuel to run on. If you don't provide it, your metabolism will slow down and you will start storing fat; that's because your body perceives you need energy but nothing is coming in. Exercising without eating is exhausting and stressful to your body, so fuel up, even if it is just a piece of fruit. If you work out in the morning and don't like eating a full meal before doing so, switch breakfast with your morning snack; that is, eat breakfast after you get your sweat on to replenish yourself, and eat your snack before exercising. Sometimes fruit is an appropriate snack before a workout, and sometimes grains are better—it all depends on your specific prescription. But the one thing I don't want you to do is exercise on an empty stomach.

4. YOU WILL EAT REAL FOOD.

Choose your foods from the sea, land, or sky, not the factory. These are the foods you need to eat to invoke a change in your body. Change comes not from macronutrients (protein, carbs, fat) but from the thousands of micronutrients in the foods you choose—micronutrients like amino acids and minerals, all the B-vitamins and antioxidant vitamins like C and E, and the many different compounds in plants like flavonoids and carotenoids, such as lutein, zeaxanthin, and lycopene. Processed foods are largely bereft of these micronutrients, especially compared to whole ones.

5. YOU WILL DRINK HALF YOUR BODY WEIGHT IN OUNCES OF SPRING WATER EVERY DAY, WITH A MAXIMUM OF 100 OUNCES PER DAY.

This is absolutely critical to helping detoxify your body and working in conjunction with your prescription, so drink up! Don't have any other beverages until you've finished your water for the day.

For Coffee, Tea, Wine, Beer, and Cocktail Drinkers

A note about alcohol and caffeine, for those of you who frequently indulge: Both alcohol and caffeine influence insulin output, glucose metabolism, and liver function. In fact, they can interfere with an important phase of liver detoxification—so much so that these substances are often used as challenges during tests for liver function. Because of this, I typically remove both of these from the diet when my goal is to get a client healthy.

6. YOU WILL REMAIN CURIOUS ABOUT YOUR BODY AND STAY IN TOUCH WITH THE SELF-DISCOVERY ZONES AND YOUR SELF-ASSESSMENT QUESTIONNAIRE AND HEALTH WISH LISTS TO MONITOR YOUR PROGRESS.

As your prescription begins to repair your metabolic pathways, keeping in touch with what symptoms you have overcome and which Health Wish List issues you have achieved will help inspire you to continue and, when necessary, to move to the next issue you want to tackle.

7. YOU WILL TELL YOUR DOCTOR YOU ARE WORKING ON YOUR ISSUE USING FOOD THERAPY, SO YOU CAN GET SUPPORT FROM YOUR DOCTOR, WHO CAN MONITOR YOUR PROGRESS AND ANY MEDICATIONS YOU MIGHT BE ON WITH THE APPROPRIATE LAB TESTS.

If you are on medication, effective food therapy could change your condition and possibly necessitate an altered dose, or even, with your doctor's approval, cessation of drug therapy when appropriate. It's important that your doctor knows what you are doing—keep everyone on your health-care team in the loop!

LET'S AGREE ON A FEW OTHER THINGS

Understanding how to take your prescription is important, but understanding how to think about your treatment is equally important. Let's agree on a few basic principles that will assist you as you restore your health.

AGREEMENT #1: YOU WILL BE GRATEFUL FOR THE STATE OF YOUR BODY RIGHT NOW.

You have a smart body. Whether you are lacking vitality, or your body has morphed into something you don't recognize, or you have a chronic disease, be grateful that your body is doing everything it possibly can to keep you alive.

AGREEMENT #2: NEVER AGAIN WILL YOU BUY INTO THE NOTION THAT LESS WILL CREATE MORE.

Food, not a lack of food, is always the solution. If you're going to hang around with me, you might as well get used to it!

AGREEMENT #3: YOUR KITCHEN IS YOUR PHARMACY.

You will mix your own prescriptions (that is, you will cook food).

If you want to benefit from food, you have to start getting into the kitchen and cooking instead of eating processed food or going out to dinner every night. Coming into the kitchen should feel like a welcome home, not like a visit to a foreign land. Cooking at home is one of the best things you can do for your health, and it doesn't have to take any longer than the time involved in waiting for a delivery or going to a restaurant. You'll also save a ton of money.

AGREEMENT #4: YOU WILL FILL YOUR FREEZER WITH FOOD YOU'VE PACKAGED, INSTEAD OF WITH PACKAGED FOOD.

Every time you cook, make extra and freeze it for later. Pretty soon, you will have a freezer full of "convenience food" that is actually good for you, that you made yourself, and that helps to heal your metabolism—and all you have to do is defrost and warm it up!

ASSEMBLING YOUR DREAM TEAM

When repairing and optimizing your health becomes a priority in your life, it is important to have a dream team of professionals to help you. This will include a primary care physician you trust and who understands and supports your health priorities. You might have or choose someone conventionally trained, or a functional medicine doctor, a naturopath, or an osteopath. Also on your team should be any specialists relevant to conditions you have (endocrinologists, cardiologists, therapists, oncologists, hematologists, orthopedists, etc.) and other health-care providers who can give you what you need or help you learn. These helpers could include massage therapists, physical or occupational therapists, acupuncturists, herbalists, homeopaths, chiropractors, or other natural or complementary health-care professionals. You may not be interested in anything but a good massage therapist, and that's fine, but if you want to learn more about some of these alternative health modalities, add experienced natural health providers to your team.

Individuals who carry titles such as naturopathic doctors, osteopathic doctors, functional medicine doctors, acupuncturists, massage therapists, neurofeedback therapists, and occupational and physical therapists are all likely to support your efforts. Keep in mind that a lot of people think they can't afford these kinds of providers, but look at your health insurance. Many plans provide for these healing modalities. I had a client who told me she couldn't afford physical therapy, but when we looked at her insurance, we realized she was covered for twenty-five physical therapy appointments every year. Become savvy about your insurance resources and support resources available to you, such as through your college, or place of employment, or a local school or university.

YOUR DOCTOR

Of course, first and foremost is your primary care doctor, who should be able to guide you and answer your questions without getting impatient or rushing you out the door. This is why it's so important to find someone you can talk to and whose beliefs are in line with yours (or at least not in opposition). It also helps to understand a little bit about how doctors think, how to talk to them, and how to ask for the tests and procedures you know you need. You are the best authority when it comes to your body, and it's your choice who plays on your team. Think of yourself as a consumer, not a patient.

The concept that food is your number-one therapy may be foreign to your doctor, who probably didn't receive a lot of nutritional training. (This is why doctors often send their clients to nutritionists—this is our specialty.) If you have a health issue, or want help in preventing one, you need your doctor. Your doctor can diagnose your health issues, run lab tests, write prescriptions, and give you good general health advice. When you and your doctor aren't on the same page, this can be a real problem.

I've been working with doctors for many years now, and I have learned some things. Here is my advice for developing a productive relationship with your doctor.

- *Ask questions.* When you know you will be seeing your doctor, write down a list of questions and make two copies. When you see your doctor, hand her or him a copy at the beginning of the appointment and ask that it be added to your file. Do not let your doctor give the paper back to you. Say, "I have a copy—that is for my file, please." Then, with your notes to give you confidence, *ask what you want to know!* If your doctor is rushing you, just ask, "Can I ask you a couple of questions that are really important to me?" A good doctor will stop talking and let you voice your concerns. Don't be afraid. No question about your health is stupid or a waste of anyone's time. If you feel rushed, ask the doctor to help you make a second appointment within that week or the next week, when she or he will have more time to talk. This will let your doctor know that you are serious about getting your questions answered and, typically, many doctors will either make the time for you right then and there, or help you set a follow-up appointment just for questions. Emphasize that the follow-up needs to be no further out than a week from your current appointment.

- *Put it in writing.* If one of your questions is to ask for a lab test, put this in writing and state the reason you believe the lab test is necessary and/or why you are requesting it (don't worry; you'll know what to ask for after reading this book; see page 258 for a sample letter). Doctors are often required to justify lab work to insurance companies, and your written request can help your doctor determine the reason to put down on the paperwork.

- *Get copies.* After you have the lab results, always ask for a copy of the results and don't leave the office without it. Many doctors' offices now have online portals where you can access your lab results 24/7, which makes this even easier. Also, when your lab tests are run and you get the results back, always bring along the list of the tests you requested. I can't tell you how many times my office has requested, for example, seven tests to be run, and then we get the results back for five of them. Make sure when your doctor's office gives you the lab request, you take your list of requested tests and the lab requisition when you go to get your blood drawn. Ask the staff at the lab to review both and make sure that every box has been checked. It is very easy for a lab to call the doctor's office and confirm an additional lab is needed, should it have been missed on the requisition. It is much more difficult to justify going back for another blood draw four to six weeks later, after the results have come in and you have discovered some of what you requested wasn't run. Keeping good records and being diligent on your own behalf can save you a lot of time, trouble, and money.

- *Keep your chart.* Get a copy of your chart and bring it with you to each doctor's appointment, even though the doctor's office keeps a copy of your chart as well. Always sit and review your chart while you're waiting for your appointment. You need to be 100 percent up to date on what's going on with your body and on what is in that chart before you walk into the examination room. You cannot ever assume that the doctor knows you as well as you know yourself, or will remember everything you've done and every test you've had run.

- *Don't ask for drugs.* Even though the commercials on national television beg to differ, do *not* walk into your doctor's office asking for a specific medication (or any medications). Ask for lab tests and other diagnostic tests, and ask for medical advice and educational knowledge about what is happening to you, but don't be in a rush to get on medication. If you really need medication, your doctor will tell you. If you don't, you are lucky and are better off tackling your issue with a food prescription and lifestyle changes. There are many undesirable and even permanently damaging side effects to medications. If you need the medicine, you need it, but this is not your ideal scenario.

- *Tell all.* Make sure you tell your doctor everything you're doing. It's okay if the two of you don't agree. A good doctor doesn't have to share your exact opinions on, for example, supplements or holistic health practices, like acupuncture. You're looking for a person who is going to bring fresh ideas to the table—ideas that maybe you haven't thought of. Your doctor is part of your health-care team, but not its leader. That's your job. If your doctor is in serious disagreement with a therapy that you're doing, ask for studies or research that back up his or her objections. If this is then provided, take that information and look at it honestly. Does your doctor's opinion fit with your model of care for your health? Maybe your doctor has a good point, and the thing you are doing isn't good for you; or, maybe your doctor doesn't understand what you are going for or is simply of a different mindset. A doctor's educated opinion is always worth considering. As you can imagine, I have strong opinions when I walk into a doctor's office, and I've chosen incredibly intelligent physicians to help me in my health journey. I welcome their opinions, even when they are in complete opposition to mine, because this gives me either a new way to look at things or a stronger conviction in the path I am taking.

- *Don't give up.* Remember the word *NO* is just an acronym for "Next Opportunity." If you try a protocol and your issue doesn't change, it's an opportunity to try something else. Ask about an alternative approach . . . and never be afraid to look for a doctor whose goals for you are more in line with your own. If your doctor tries to intimidate you out of getting the answers, tests, or treatment you know you need, you always have the right to go elsewhere.

There's a book by Egyptian writer Wael Ghonim about revolution, subtitled *The Power of the People Is Greater than the People in Power.* You are the consumer, and just as when you ask the manager of your grocery store to start carrying a product you like, you can ask your doctor to do the tests you want or to respect your preferences in treatment. I drive my doctor crazy, but

I have learned over many years as both a patient and a colleague that you have to create relationships with your caregiver. The only way to do that is to let the individual know something about you. If you don't do anything else, the next time you visit a new doctor or specialist, introduce yourself. Tell him or her something interesting about your world. Also, you can't sit by and be passive. My fifteen-year-old nephew was recently given a narcotic in a doctor's office, and nobody even asked for my sister's consent. He had an ear infection, his ear drum had ruptured, and they administered oxycodone. He wasn't in the emergency room or even in the hospital. My sister called me in a panic because when they got home, the poor kid was completely out of it.

Your doctor will not necessarily tell you everything you need or want to know, and will also not necessarily customize treatment for your individual situation. Your doctor might not even know all the details of your individual situation, if he or she hasn't run all the tests or thoroughly examined your history. I can't tell you how many clients I have—bright, intelligent people, the kind who run companies and organizations and households, who form charities and sit on boards—who are on medications and have no idea why or what the medications do. Or, how many of those same folks were on medications that negatively interacted with other meds, or that weren't suited for the client's individual manifestations of the health issue.

It can be difficult to talk to a doctor who isn't hearing you, and it can be difficult to stand up for yourself when you aren't an expert and you don't have all the information. But you must put yourself back into the equation (the "me" in metabolism), and that means taking 100 percent responsibility for communicating any health issue to your doctor. To do that, you need information, and that's what I'm giving you in this book—the tools and resources to put yourself in charge of your health. Don't be afraid to have your lab tests run. If you have a disease, you need to know what you can do to give your body every chance of healing. If you have a predisposition to a health condition, you need to know the best way to prevent its happening to you. That's power, not helplessness.

Don't let anything or anyone define or dictate how healthy you can be.

LISTENING TO YOUR BODY IN THE LAB

Another very important thing a doctor can do for you is to order lab tests. I utilize the lab frequently with my clients because, although you know your own body better than anyone else, lab tests can give unique insights into where things are getting out of balance. You might think you feel just fine (especially if you aren't yet accustomed to listening to your body) and not realize that cholesterol is pooling in your blood or your blood sugars are too high, or any number of other small changes that can happen in your body; a lab test can help to reveal and validate.

Many of my clients go to the doctor for a physical exam and some basic lab tests. Although it's not required—because through self-discovery and self-assessment we can forge a clear path—it is an option for you. If you want to establish a baseline of health and you want to know test results, go ahead and have those done before you begin, or at any time during the process. A baseline check-up and some standard tests to measure your health right now will give you the means to monitor how well you are doing on your nutritional prescription. If you are working to metabolize cholesterol more efficiently, for example, you'll get to see where your cholesterol numbers are at an initial test and then see them go down after a repeated test once you've completed your first month's prescription. Then you get to watch them go down even more with every monthly test, until your cholesterol is right where you and your doctor want it to be (in other words, until your body is *metabolizing cholesterol properly*).

Although your doctor may recommend some additional tests depending on your physical examination, these are the general tests I recommend all clients do at least once every year, to keep track of what is going on inside and to best tailor nutritional prescriptions and lifestyle activities. These tests are all likely covered on health insurance policies as part of a basic yearly physical examination, but be sure to tell your doctor all your symptoms so he or she can justify any additional tests your insurance company might not automatically cover:

- **Complete blood count (CBC):** This test is often used as a general health check. It looks at your red and white blood cell counts and other components of your blood. Abnormal results can indicate many different things, so this is a level-one screening that any doctor should be happy to perform at an annual physical.

- **Blood chemistry:** This test screens your blood for a wide range of substances that could be abnormally present or absent if you are having health issues. This is a very general test, but is a good way to catch problems before they go too far.

- **Liver panel:** This is a series of tests that checks for any abnormal liver values and can indicate if your liver is overburdened or not functioning as it should.

- **Lipid panel:** This test looks at different kinds of fat in your blood. It checks your cholesterol levels, including HDL, LDL, and triglycerides. More advanced lipid tests break down cholesterol into even more categories, for further investigation of cholesterol or lipid issues that could signify heart disease risk or presence.

- **Hemoglobin A1C:** This test is useful to detect unstable blood sugar levels or potential problems with the interaction between blood sugar and insulin, which can occur in prediabetic conditions.

- **C-reactive protein (CRP):** This test measures inflammation in the body.

FOUNDATIONAL MOVEMENT

The human body is meant to move. It is specifically constructed to walk, run, jump, swim, lift, and carry. Being able to move is an important part of keeping the human body functioning. As I do with my clients, the kind of movement I want you to incorporate into your life (if you haven't already) depends on what's going on with you. It depends on what you are eating, what your environment is like, what health issues you have, and what metabolic pathways we are attempting to rebalance.

For each of the nutritional prescriptions in this book, I will give you a particular movement prescription. Foundationally, however, all I ask is that you incorporate movement into your daily life. This might be active movement (like walking) or passive movement (like massage). It might be vigorous movement (like a spin class) or gentle movement (like stretching.) Choose what movement feels good to you, but be sure it meets these requirements:

- It should not hurt. Pain encourages dysfunctional metabolic pathways.

- It should not exhaust you. Exhaustion encourages dysfunction in metabolic pathways.

- It should not be overstimulating and negatively stressful. Negative stress encourages dysfunctional metabolic pathways. If you are exercising like an athlete, you must feed yourself like an athlete. There has to be a balance between the way in which you push your body and the way in which you nurture it.

- Exercising for metabolic repair (as opposed to training for a competition, for example) should not make you feel ill—nauseated, headachy, or as if you have a fever or swollen lymph glands, either during or afterwards. These are all signs that you are utilizing a dysfunctional metabolic pathway and overly stressing your body.

If your movement of choice does any of these things—causes pain, exhaustion, or overstimulation, or makes you feel ill in any way—then it isn't right for you at this point in your life, as you are seeking to heal your metabolism. It is not the right movement for you now.

Maybe you've just signed up for a spin class or you are planning to train for a marathon, but the thought fills you with dread, or your first class or training session is painful, exhausting, or makes you feel sick or stressed. That isn't the right movement for you now. Pharmaceutical labels sometimes have warnings like: *Do not operate heavy machinery or drive until you know how this prescription affects you.* Consider your movement prescription to be like that: until you have oriented yourself in your new way of eating and living, be gentle with your movements and fit them into your life in a way that feels good, not bad.

READING AND WRITING YOUR MEAL MAPS

Meal maps are an integral part of my practice, and I give them to all my clients. A meal map is simply a template that organizes your meals for you. Every nutritional prescription in this book has its unique meal map, so when you get to yours, I want you to understand what it is, how it works, and how to use it.

The meal maps in this book look like tables, with columns for breakfast, lunch, dinner, and snacks. For some of the nutritional prescriptions, you will eat five times each day; for others, you will add an evening snack for a total of six times per day.

Within each meal, the meal map will tell you what *type of food* to put into that slot. For example, your particular prescription for breakfast might look like this:

BREAKFAST
Complex Carbs
Fruit
Healthy Fat

This means that for that particular prescription, for that meal, you should choose a whole grain, a fruit, and a healthy fat for your meal, from the Foundational Foods List at the end of this chapter (and highlighting the foods you will find on the special Top 20 Power Foods lists, which are subsets of the Foundational Foods List specifically targeted for each prescription).

An important thing for you to understand as you choose the foods you want to fill out your meal map is this:

> In Chapters 5 through 11, your specific nutritional prescription is a combination of strategic foods (especially those on the Top 20 Power Foods list for your prescription, but also from the Foundational Foods List) and strategically timed and positioned foods at each meal. This is what brings metabolic repair. I want you to eat from the Foundational Foods List, giving special attention to the Top 20 Power Foods, but the power foods are not the entire prescription, by any means. Follow the meal map, fill it in with the power foods and foundational foods, and you will be doing everything correctly.

These lists are your most valuable tools. They are so important because they contain many healthful whole foods with micronutrients specifically appropriate for metabolic repair. They are also important because they don't contain: metabolism-dampening foods, or foods known to cause issues, or foods that contribute to interference with any of the metabolic pathways we are working on clearing. For example, the Foundational Foods List includes wild-caught salmon but not bologna, the latter of which is full of chemical additives. The list includes oranges but not orange juice, because orange juice has a glycemic index (G.I.) that is too high and can raise your blood sugar too quickly. The list includes brown rice pasta but not wheat pasta, as wheat pasta causes an inflammatory reaction in many people.

For this breakfast example, you would not choose anything beyond what is on the list. You might have sprouted-grain toast with almond butter and a bowl of blueberries, or oatmeal with sliced peaches and coconut milk, but you wouldn't add turkey bacon (for example) because protein is not on the list.

In this way, you get to choose what you like, but you eat only the components of that meal as they are prescribed for you. Chapters 5 through 11 show one sample day with some recipes that fit your particular prescriptive meal map. This is meant to get you started and show you how to incorporate the right foods at the right time. The goal is to use the meal map to enjoy the foods you like. Get creative. You can even adapt your favorite recipes to fit your prescription. If you need more inspiration, you can find many more recipes on my website, www.hayliepomroy.com. We will be continually adding resources for you on the website, so visit often. We are there for you!

THE FOUNDATIONAL FOODS LIST

This list of foundational foods is the list from which you should make your primary dietary choices. I have developed this list over years of clinical practice, so you can be assured that it contains the most nutrient-dense and metabolically useful foods that nature makes available to us. If you eat from this list most of the time, you will help shore up your body's micronutrient reserves and give it everything it needs to create energy, bone, and muscle—and to mend the body.

This is a great list of food choices for everyone, but it is particularly critical when you are following one of my nutritional prescriptions. Every nutritional prescription I write for you in this book will use foods from this list. In essence, this is the pharmacy from which you will fill your nutritional prescriptions. Its micronutrients create a healthy and vigorous metabolism and contribute to both repair and restoration.

Some of the foods on this list have special qualities targeted for specific issues. That is why, for each nutritional prescription in the following seven chapters, you will also find a list of the Top 20 Power Foods for that condition, derived from this Foundational Foods List. These power foods are most specifically and strategically appropriate for addressing particular issues. Any whole food has a complex profile of macronutrients, micronutrients, and phytonutrients, and these interact with other whole foods in unique ways as they are combined or consumed at different times of the day. As you fill out your meal maps, favor these power foods as much as you can, but also choose from other foods on the Foundational Foods List to fill in the gaps and make your meals enjoyable and satisfying. Eating this way, you will be feeding your body, healing your metabolism, and nourishing the metabolic pathways to help your body regain its balance.

But in case you are looking for nutrient information, understand that this is not a reference for the nutritional contents of individual foods and what they can do. To me, such references reflect a simplistic and reductionist approach that doesn't capture the innate complexity of the human body or the way the metabolism uses food. We are focusing here on repairing specific metabolic pathways with a variety of effective approaches that I have combined in my own practice, in a way that has shown to work.

There are multiple food philosophies evident in the construction of this list and these prescriptions. To invoke clinical change, I pull from the philosophies of food combining, elimination and rotation diets, meal timing, modification of glycemic values, protein rotation, and, yes, targeted micronutrients. But here, these philosophies are all used together to create a nutrition plan that can bring about metabolic change. So don't look for simplistic "this nutrient = that magical disease fix." Instead of worrying whether vitamin X does Y, follow me into the fascinating world of food as medicine, and watch your body transform as this Foundational Foods List becomes your medicine chest.

HOW TO USE THE FOOD LISTS

These are the foods that will form the foundation of your daily diet. They can be eaten in any of the plans to help you follow your specific nutritional prescriptions. Even if you have none of the health issues discussed in this book, and just want a healthy foundation for eating, choose from this list. It is your go-to source for health.

VEGETABLES
SERVING SIZE: UNLIMITED

Alfalfa sprouts

Artichokes—all types, fresh, frozen, jarred, or canned without additives, not marinated. Artichokes and water should be the only ingredients stated on package.

Arugula

Asparagus

Bamboo shoots

Beans—green, yellow wax, haricots verts

Bean sprouts

Beets—fresh or canned, no sugar added

Beets—greens and bulbs

Bok choy

Broccoli

Broccolini

Brussels sprouts

Cabbage—all types, including fermented/cultured, such as sauerkraut and kimchi

Carrots

Cauliflower

Celery—including leaves

Chicory—especially curly endive

Collard greens

Cucumbers—all types

Cultured/fermented veggies—all types, such as sauerkraut, kimchi, and cultured pickles

Daikon (white radish)

Dandelion greens

Eggplant

Endive

Fennel

Frisée

Hearts of palm

Jícama

Kale

Leafy greens (mixed)

Leeks

Lettuces—all types except iceberg

Mushrooms

Mustard greens

Okra

Onions—red, yellow, green (scallions)

Parsnips

Peppers—sweet and hot: Anaheim, banana, cherry, habanero, jalapeño, pepperoncini, poblano, and serrano chiles; bell, Italian frying, pimiento sweet peppers

Pumpkin

Radishes

Rhubarb

Rutabaga

Sea vegetable/seaweeds—dulse, hijiki, kelp, kombu, nori

Shallots

Snow peas

Spinach

Spirulina (type of algae)

Sprouts—all types

Summer squash—yellow, zucchini

Swiss chard

Turnips

Watercress

Winter squash—acorn, butternut, delicata, pumpkin, spaghetti squash

FRUITS (all fruits and vegetables can be fresh or frozen, unless otherwise noted)
SERVING SIZE: 1 CUP OR 1 PIECE

Low glycemic fruits (0–49)

Apples—all types

Blackberries

Blueberries

Cherries

Goji berries

Grapefruit

Kumquats

Lemons

Limes

Loganberries

Mulberries

Oranges

Peaches

Pears—all types

Plums

Prickly pears

Prunes

Strawberries

Tomatoes (for our purposes, tomatoes are fruit, not vegetable)

High glycemic fruits (50–100)

Apricots

Cantaloupe

Clementine

Cranberries

Figs—fresh only

Guavas

Honeydew melon

Kiwi

Mangos

Nectarines

Papayas

Pineapple

Pomegranates

Raspberries

Tangerines

Watermelon

COMPLEX CARBS
SERVING SIZE: 1 CUP COOKED GRAIN; ½ CUP COOKED LEGUMES;
1 OUNCE CRACKERS OR PRETZELS; 1 SLICE BREAD; 1 TORTILLA; ½ BAGEL;
1 MEDIUM SWEET POTATO

Amaranth

Barley—black or white

Beans/legumes—white, black, kidney, lima, pinto, adzuki; no peanuts, peas or soybeans

Brown rice pasta

Buckwheat flour

Kamut flour/bagels

Freekah (a green wheat that is roasted; considered an "ancient grain")

Millet

Nut flours

Oats/oatmeal

Quinoa

Rice—brown, black, red, wild

Rye flour

Sorghum

Spelt—pasta, pretzels, tortillas

Sprouted-grain bagels, breads, tortillas

Sweet potatoes/yams (for our purposes, sweet potatoes and yams are complex carbs, not vegetables)

Tapioca, as a thickener in recipes (not the pudding with added sugar)

Teff

Wheat grass (serving size one shot)

PROTEINS

Animal Protein SERVING SIZE: 4 OUNCES MEAT OR 6 OUNCES FISH

Beef—all lean cuts, lean ground meat, rump roast

Buffalo

Calamari

Caviar

Chicken

Clams

Corned beef

Crab meat

Cured lean meats—prosciutto, black forest ham, smoked ham (only if nitrate free)

Deli meats—turkey, chicken, roast beef (only if nitrate free)

Eggs, whole, any size (2 eggs make a serving)

Fish—wild-caught, any types, especially cod, dory, flounder, haddock, halibut, herring, mackerel, pollock, sardines, sea bass, skate, sole, and trout (avoid bottom feeders, which tend to be more polluted, such as tilapia, grouper, and catfish)

Game—venison, elk, pheasant, etc.

Guinea fowl

Jerky—beef, buffalo, turkey, elk, ostrich

Lamb

Lobster

Mussels

Organ meats—chicken liver or gizzards, beef liver or heart, sweetbreads, kidneys, etc.

Oysters, fresh, raw or cooked; or packaged, packed in water

Pork—tenderloin, loin roast, chops

Rabbit

Salmon—smoked, fresh, frozen, or canned

Scallops

Shrimp

Tuna—fresh, frozen, or canned

Turkey

Vegetarian Protein SERVING SIZE: ½ CUP COOKED LEGUMES/COOKED MUSHROOMS; ½ CUP COOKED GRAINS; ¼ CUP RAW NUTS

Note: Some items on this list also appear on other lists, such as the Complex Carbs, Vegetables, or Healthy Fats lists. These foods can be used for either purpose in your meal map, but serving sizes will vary depending on how you are using them.

Almond cheese/almond flour

Beans/legumes—white, black, pinto, chickpeas, lentils, adzuki, etc.; no peanuts, peas, or soybeans

Mushrooms

Nuts and seeds—raw only, all types (almond, Brazil, chia, pecan, pumpkin, sesame, walnuts, etc.), including their butters

Oat bran

Quinoa

Rye berries

Wild rice

HEALTHY FATS
SERVING SIZE: 1 CUP NUT MILKS; ¼ CUP RAW NUTS AND SEEDS OR
SHREDDED COCONUT; ¼ CUP OLIVES; 3 TABLESPOONS DRESSING;
2 TABLESPOONS OIL; 2 TABLESPOONS RAW NUT OR SEED BUTTERS

Almond milk

Avocado—½ medium

Cashew milk

Coconut

Coconut milk

Coconut oil

Flaxseed

Grapeseed oil

Hummus (⅓ cup)

Mayonnaise—safflower oil based

Olive oil

Olives

Nuts and seeds—raw only, all types
(almond, Brazil, chia, pecan, pumpkin,
sesame, walnuts, etc.), including their
butters

Sesame oil

Tahini (sesame butter)

HERBS, SPICES, CONDIMENTS, AND MISCELLANEOUS FOODS
SERVING SIZE: UNLIMITED

Agar agar

Apple cider vinegar

Arrowroot powder

Black pepper

Broths and stocks, homemade or
natural/sugar-free—beef, chicken,
vegetable, turkey

Cacao powder, raw

Chili powder

Chives

Coconut aminos

Dried or fresh herbs—basil, bay
leaf, celery seed, dill, mint, oregano,
parsley, rosemary, tarragon, thyme
(note: all peppers, including spices
from chiles, such as red pepper flakes
and cayenne, are to be avoided when
on the autoimmune prescription)

Garlic—fresh, and garlic powder

Ginger, fresh or ground

Horseradish, fresh or jarred

Lemon peel, lemon verbena leaves

Lime peel

Mustard—all types

Nutritional yeast

Pickles

Salsa, including fermented

Sea salt

Sesame seeds

Spices—cinnamon, coriander, cumin,
turmeric, nutmeg

Spices from peppers—cayenne
pepper, chili powder, red pepper
flakes, paprika, etc.

Sweeteners—pure stevia or birch-
based xylitol

Tabasco

Tamari

Vanilla extract

Vinegars—any type (including
coconut vinegar and rice vinegar
as long as it doesn't contain added
sugar)

Xanthan gum (non-corn-based)

About Smoothies and Juices

I am a big advocate of smoothies, but I am not an advocate of juicing—and here's why: I want you to eat *whole* food, and juices are not whole foods. Smoothies are a whole food that is pureed, and purees can be a delicious and more digestible way to get your vegetables and fruits. Juices, however, remove the fiber and also concentrate the sugars in vegetables and fruits, which can cause blood sugar instability. The only time I do not advocate eating whole foods is when certain micronutrients are used therapeutically in supplement form. In my life and in the life of my clients, supplements have brought about real clinical change without concentrating sugars in the body. So blend all the smoothies you desire, but maybe keep that juicer in the pantry.

Now you are prepared to choose your nutritional prescription. If you already know which issue you want to address first, jump right in. If you aren't sure, read the next seven chapters. Each chapter features a Self-Discovery Zone that pinpoints some of the ways your body may be whispering, talking, or screaming a message. See which messages are most familiar to you. Be curious! In Chapter 12, you will find a Whole-Body Diagnosis Quiz to help you discover where your body might be suggesting you begin; that may be all you need to figure out where to start.

If you have more than one of these health issues, begin with the one that bothers you the most—or, alternatively, start at the very beginning with the GI chapter, and work your way through them, one at a time. All of these prescriptions will be beneficial, therapeutic, and metabolically healing, so you can't go wrong.

Your body can do amazing things. Every breath you take and every bite of food you consume are new opportunities to heal, balance, or potentially clean a metabolic pathway. Remember: Everything you do has the potential to create health, just as it has to create imbalance. No matter how far down the wrong path you have wandered, it is never too late to make that U-turn.

Go Raw and Soak

Nuts and seeds are some of my favorite healthy snacks. They contain the kind of fat that encourages fat burning and have nutrients that feed some of your most important metabolic pathways. However, only eat raw nuts and seeds that have been soaked.

Roasted nuts may taste good to you because you are used to them, but they can contain added fat and chemicals called acrylamides that form during the roasting process and that are carcinogenic. Raw nuts and seeds don't contain these substances; they do, however, contain phytic acid, which can block the body's absorption of the nut's nutrients. To get rid of the phytic acid and to generate useful enzymes inside the nuts and seeds, you soak them before eating. Here's how: Put your nuts or seeds in a glass jar and cover with purified water. Put them in the refrigerator for 24 hours. Drain, rinse, dry, and store in ¼ cup serving sizes in sealed plastic bags in the fridge for up to a week or freezer for up to two months. Easy snacks!

If you want to achieve health, you need to eat foods that support your metabolism! Every day, ask yourself: "Did I Eat Today (D.I.E.T.) to accomplish my health goals?"

When it comes to food, I know what I'm talking about. I can help you. Use me. Use my expertise. I can empower you to make good health happen to you. And along with good health, I can give you the body you want, in the size and shape you want, at the weight you want. I can help you perform better in sports, in the bedroom, in life. I can optimize you.

Let me do that! Pick your health issues, then check them off your to-do list so you never have to think of them again. Let's get started!

PART TWO

Your Body Is Whispering

CHAPTER 5

Gastrointestinal Dysfunction, Indigestion, and IBS

Every time you eat, there is a process that allows that food to enter your system and that allows your body to digest and metabolize the food, transforming it into energy and nutrients your body can use to heal, rebuild, and re-create itself. Because metabolism is the conversion of food into fuel and action, and because digestion is the process through which we absorb food into our body's internal ecosystem, think of your gastrointestinal (GI) tract as the ultimate gatekeeper. If food is medicine, and you can't process the food, you can't get the medicine you need to address any of the problems described in this book. Any prescription from here on out, then, is *nutrient dependent*; if you can't receive the nutrients, you can't reap the benefits.

Your gastrointestinal tract is your mode of delivery for this powerful medicine. Imagine if you needed an injectable medication but you didn't have a needle or a syringe. That medication would be useless. Imagine if you had an oral medication but you refused to open your mouth. That medication would be useless. In the same way, the nutrient-dependent prescriptions I give you won't work if your body isn't digesting, assimilating, and absorbing food as well as it can—or eliminate the waste as well as it should. Your GI tract is your body's first interaction with the food you eat. It is the front line, where you protect yourself from what is harmful and you mobilize to use what is beneficial. It simply *has* to work.

But as with any system in the body, sometimes things go wrong—and when it comes to digestion, things often go wrong. In fact, it is estimated that one in six people in the United States, or almost 50 million of us, suffer from irritable bowel syndrome (IBS),[14] a common condition that makes constipation, diarrhea, stomach cramps, gas, and bloating regular events associated with eating.[15] Many others suffer from some form of indigestion, like acid reflux or heartburn. Some suffer from small intestinal bacterial overgrowth (SIBO), or a proliferation of bacteria in the small intestine that should be in the colon, or structural dysfunctions like diverticulitis.

Digestive diseases can become severe. When the immune system gets involved, conditions like celiac disease can damage the gastrointestinal tract, flattening and killing the tiny hairs, called villi, that absorb the nutrients from the food you eat. Chronic serious conditions like Crohn's disease and other forms of inflammatory bowel disease (IBD) can cause extreme discomfort, leading you to feel they have taken over your life.

But in many cases, digestive complaints can seem relatively mild. They are whispers. You may just pop an over-the-counter remedy for your heartburn or constipation, and figure that it's no big deal. Some of the most common and most purchased over-the-counter medications target such digestive issues; in fact, people take more antacids, antigas products, laxatives, stool softeners, and diarrhea remedies than any other over-the-counter medication.[16] When you have these kinds of problems, especially IBS and indigestion or bloating or gas after eating, your body is whispering to you that something is out of balance. If you ignore those whispers, the message will get louder and louder. By the time you've developed an autoimmune condition like celiac disease or an extreme case of inflammatory bowel disease like Crohn's, they will have turned into a scream. In other words, *ignore those whispers at your peril.*

When there is an imbalance in the GI tract—for instance, something gets in that causes a reaction, such as an allergen or virus, or the body is unable to fully metabolize or utilize the nutrients from food, including fat, protein, sugar, or micronutrients—this can trigger a disease process. Nutrient deficiency as a result of absorption issues can introduce a host of other problems, including:

- The improper repair and rebuilding of bone and muscle

- Poor organ maintenance

- Problems in the body's detoxification system

- The proper release of hormones that govern most bodily processes

- The balance of gut bacteria that influences mood

- The body's likelihood of launching an attack on itself and developing an autoimmune disease like rheumatoid arthritis

- The body's tendency to hoard fat rather than burn it

Gastrointestinal dysfunction may be *the first sign that something is going wrong*, even if it isn't the first step in a chain reaction happening inside your body. Your body isn't handling the food you eat the way it should, and that can set off a chain reaction of health issues that become increasingly difficult to resolve. Remember: The nature and health of your internal ecosystem determines whether the nutrients from food you eat, the digestive enzymes produced by your organs, and the serotonin produced in your gut can each do what they need to do. If you want real healing and true health, you can't just take a laxative and call it a day.

THE SELF-DISCOVERY ZONE

You may not know for sure what the nature of your gastrointestinal issues is, but your body knows and it is trying to tell you. Here are some of the symptoms you might be experiencing that can help you determine whether you are having digestive issues. These symptoms might come from food reactivity, insufficient enzyme production, or a gut flora imbalance, but no matter the underlying cause, your body is whispering to you: "Hey, not all is well with the digestion down here! Can you do something about it?"

- Acid reflux or heartburn after eating or after going too long without eating

- Allergy shiners—those dark puffy circles under the eyes

- Asthma

- Bloating after eating, even to the extent of looking pregnant

- Bowel movements that come out in long, thin ropes

- Cellulite that develops suddenly and in large amounts

- Frequent colds or other viral infections

- Congestion or stuffy nose after eating

- Dry or blotchy skin

- Eczema

- Eyelash thickening for no apparent reason (this sounds like a good thing, but especially in kids, it is actually a sign of food reactivity)

- Food allergies

- Frequent canker sores

- Frequent constipation or diarrhea (or alternating between the two)

- Gas and flatulence

- Lipomas (little fat pockets in strange places, such as under the eyelids)

- Nails and hair that become weaker and thinner

- Painful joints or a diagnosis of arthritis

- Rash on the backs of your arms

- Rectal itching

- Saddlebags or other fat accumulation in areas you didn't have before

- Skin rashes that are frequent and unexplained, that could occur anywhere from face to feet

- Stomach pains or a "nervous stomach"

- Undigested food in your stool

- Yeast infections that recur frequently

If any of these sound familiar, you probably have some form of gastrointestinal dysfunction, including IBS or indigestion or both. Your body wants your attention, and it is sending you a clear message. Let's give your body what it really needs—right now.

DEALING, NOT HEALING

Gastrointestinal or digestive disorders are among the most common complaints heard in doctors' offices and also in emergency rooms. Doctors hear a lot about stomach pain, gas and bloating, heartburn and acid reflux, constipation, diarrhea, and nausea. Digestive issues are even sometimes mistaken for heart attacks. With such a widespread problem, you would think we all would go for the easy and obvious solution (changing what we eat); but instead, doctors tend to prescribe medication. For example, indigestion, heartburn, and acid reflux are typically treated with drugs that block acid production, such as proton pump inhibitors like Prevacid, Prilosec, and Nexium. Never mind that proton pump inhibitors can increase your risk of diabetes, and are also a risk to your heart!

Other drugs block acid. Called H2 blockers, these include medications like Pepcid, Zantac, and Tagamet. Constipation is typically treated with laxatives or fiber supplements, even though chemical laxatives can really mess up your electrolyte balance and can even lead to heart disturbances. For peptic ulcers, the typical treatment includes antibiotics along with more acid-blocking medication.

In other words, drugs are the conventional answer to these conditions. Some doctors might mention that you could take a fiber supplement, but beyond that, you probably won't get any lifestyle advice. You might even be told that your condition is one you will just have to live with, and all you can really do is try to control your symptoms. Hogwash.

TARGETED PATHWAYS FOR REPAIR

There is a whole school of thought that says digestion is the root of all health, and that without healing the gut, you cannot heal any disease. There is a lot of merit to this point of view because, as I've explained, when your digestion isn't working you may not be absorbing nutrients well and that may impede the work of other functions to some extent. I don't always agree that digestion is the first issue everybody should tackle, though—sometimes there are more pressing matters to get under control first. If you are having a health crisis, like diabetes or autoimmunity, you may want to start there. Yet, if we were all interfacing with food correctly, people might not ever develop high

Your gut contains 100 trillion microbes, and those microbes contain ten times more cells than you have in the rest of your entire body. These gut microbes are now known to affect the metabolism in major ways, from the body's ability to process various foods to hormone regulation, to the strength of the immune system itself. Gut microbes have even been shown to influence behavior and food preferences!* A 2013 study published in *Science* demonstrated that "microbial exposures and sex hormones exert potent effects on autoimmune diseases, many of which are more prevalent in women." The study demonstrated that "early-life microbial exposures determine sex hormone levels and modify progression to autoimmunity" in mouse models. The microbiome also determines how well you can absorb the micronutrients from the food you eat. According to a 2009 study in *Science Translational Medicine*, "The nutritional value of food is influenced in part by a person's gut microbial community (microbiota) and its component genes (microbiome)," and the content of a body's microbial community can shift significantly in a very short time based on dietary changes. In other words, the bacterial content of your digestive tract directly impacts your health in multiple ways, the significance of which science is only beginning to understand.

The good news is that we already know we can change the composition of our gut bacteria through food, nurturing those bacteria that are useful and health promoting, and making a less hospitable environment for those gut bacteria that promote disease and nudge us toward less nutritious food choices. In fact, the gut bacteria can change significantly just 24 hours after a dietary change.

---

* J. Alcock et al., "Is Eating Behavior Manipulated by the Gastrointestinal Microbiota? Evolutionary Pressure and Potential Mechanisms," *Bioessays* 36, no. 10 (October 2014): 940–49. L. A. David et al., "Diet Rapidly and Reproducibly Alters the Human Gut Microbiome," *Nature* 23 (January 2014); 505, 559–63.

cholesterol, hypertension, heart disease, diabetes, fatty pockets where we don't want them, or mood disorders like depression and anxiety. If we were all interfacing with the right foods at the right times, we probably wouldn't have bodies that morph into something we don't recognize. Remember that disease, as well as undesirable changes in body shape, are *metabolic adaptations* to the internal environment, and our interface with food is a major factor in establishing that environment.

How is your body metabolizing food? How are health issues manifesting themselves as your body's metabolic adaptations for digesting food more or less effectively? This is what I want to consider as you explore these interesting questions: *How is your digestion? Is it happening quickly enough, or too quickly? Are you reacting in a negative way to something you ate? Did you eat too much, or too little?*

For this nutritional prescription, we target the primary mechanisms of the gastrointestinal tract and its very important functions: digesting, absorbing, assimilating, and eliminating food. Specifically, we focus on:

1. **Enzyme secretion.** Enzymes are the catalysts for biochemical reactions in the body, specifically (as they relate to this chapter) the ones that extract nutrients from the foods we eat and transform them into forms the body can use to heal, repair, rebuild, and re-create itself. Enzymes are produced throughout the GI tract and by various organs, so there are many pathways that control their production and secretion, and there are different enzymes responsible for digesting different kinds of food—carbohydrates and sugars, proteins and fats, and many subcategories within those broader categories.

2. **Tissue health.** The microvilli in the small intestine and the mucosal lining that lines the entire gastrointestinal tract must be strong and healthy for proper nutrient absorption. The movement in the digestive tract itself is also an important part of tissue health. If you don't have good muscular action in the GI tract, you may have trouble eliminating waste, which can back up the entire system.

3. **Microbiome population.** The microbiome is the ecosystem of the gut. Your GI tract contains billions of bacteria that act in thousands of ways to promote health, from enzyme secretion and nutrient absorption to mood balancing and appetite control. In many ways, we are products of the bacteria in our gut, so it is extremely important to nurture bacterial populations that benefit health.

REMOVE, REPAIR, AND RESTORE

To most efficiently nurture and heal the targeted pathways for repair, we focus on foods that encourage enzyme secretion and healthy bacteria in the microbiome, as well as those that are most conducive to reducing irritation to and encouraging healing of the tissues of the gastrointestinal tract. These are our objectives:

1. Remove potential stressors to the digestive system, including reactive foods and unfriendly gut flora such as bacteria, parasites, or yeast.

2. Repair any damage to the mucosal lining of the GI tract, including the microvilli and secretory cells, and re-inoculate the gut with healthy bacteria.

3. Restore healthy elimination of toxins and food waste by encouraging healthy bowel function.

THE LOWDOWN ON FECAL IMPLANTS

It sounds like a bad joke—getting somebody else's feces implanted in your colon?—but it is not just a trendy new treatment; it's also a highly effective one for serious bacterial infections like *Clostridium difficile*, and even for weight loss among those who can afford such therapies. It's also been experimentally used to treat irritable bowel syndrome and certain neurological diseases like Parkinson's. Although it is still cutting-edge treatment, fecal pills and transplants may someday become a standard treatment for all kinds of gastrointestinal disorders.

A. Anathaswamy, "Fecal Transplant Eases Symptoms of Parkinson's," *New Scientist* 106 (January 19, 2011): S352.

GUIDELINES FOR YOUR GASTROINTESTINAL REPAIR RX

To follow your GI prescription correctly, be sure to eat exactly according to the plan, and stick to these parameters:

- You will be taking this prescription six times per day (eating six times per day). In other words, you will have three strategic, GI-balancing meals and three targeted energy-balancing snacks each day, and you will take your prescription (eat) every three to four hours during waking hours.

- To restore the ecosystem to balance and completely heal the mucosal lining, many of my clients use this prescription for six to eight months. Symptom relief is often achieved in the first two months, but the symptoms quickly come back if the support is removed too early; that's because not enough time has been allowed for new growth and healthy tissue regeneration. So stick with this plan for the long term if you want to effect lasting gastrointestinal repair.

- If you have a problem with any food on this plan, such as allergies or just plain dislike (and especially if you have any kind of individual digestive reaction to it), substitute it for any other food on the Top 20 Power Foods for GI Repair list first, and then the Foundational Foods List if you still haven't found the substitution you like best. For example, you could switch carrots for green beans or lentils for pumpkin seeds.

- Tell your doctor that you are using diet to work on your GI issues. Your doctor will likely be open to this—with or without complementary drug therapy, if that is necessary for immediate symptom relief. Your doctor might want to do some tests, but also ask for the tests I discuss at the end of this chapter for a clearer picture of where you are and to monitor your progress.

- Always travel with your food lists and meal maps. You can copy them and keep them in your purse or car, or take a picture of them with your phone. That way, you will always know what targeted digestive food to eat, even when you are out.

- Don't forget to drink half your body weight in ounces of spring water every day, with a maximum of 100 ounces per day.

EAT YOUR MEDICINE: YOUR GASTROINTESTINAL REPAIR RX

Follow this prescription precisely for best results—don't skip any meals or snacks, even if you aren't hungry. First, here is your list of Top 20 Power Foods:

TOP 20 POWER FOODS FOR GI REPAIR

These foods, excerpted from the Foundational Foods List, are your go-to food choices as you fill out your meal maps. These foods are specifically targeted to your gastrointestinal repair prescription, so use them whenever you have the opportunity.

Basil

Carrots

Celery

Coconut oil

Cultured/fermented cabbage (such as kimchi and sauerkraut)

Fennel

Green apples

Green beans

Lentils (ideally sprouted)

Mint

Pears

Pine nuts

Prunes

Raw pumpkin seeds

Red cabbage

Rosemary

Salmon

Sweet potatoes

Zucchini

For the meal map, emphasize simple meals with digestible elements to soothe the irritation; choose foods that are easy to digest for better nutrient absorption, and that encourage the colon to move everything along. This plan also encourages the proliferation of good gut bacteria and avoids common allergens.

Note that we don't focus on healthy fats in this prescription. It's okay to cook with oils that are on the Foundational Foods List. High-fat foods, though, even those with healthy fats, can be hard for a stressed gastrointestinal tract to process.

MEAL MAP FOR GI REPAIR, DAYS 1–7

BREAKFAST	SNACK	LUNCH	SNACK	DINNER	SNACK
Fruit (high or low G.I.) Healthy Fat	Vegetable (cooked)	Complex Carb Protein Vegetable	Vegetable (cooked)	Complex Carb Protein Vegetable (preferably cooked)	Fruit (cooked, high or low G.I.)

A DAY IN THE LIFE OF GI REPAIR

Now let's explore how you can implement this prescription. Here is a sample day of eating using foods from both the Top 20 Power Foods for GI Repair list and the Foundational Foods List, with a special emphasis on the power foods. I've also included recipes for one sample day, just to get you started. The recipes provided appear in boldface type in the meal map sample.

SAMPLE DAY FOR GI REPAIR, DAYS 1–7

BREAKFAST	SNACK	LUNCH	SNACK	DINNER	SNACK
Green Apple with Almond Butter	Cooked green beans	**Quinoa Crab Salad**	Cooked broccoli	**Cod with Sweet Mash and Greens**	Cooked peaches

RECIPES

In each of the recipes for this prescription, I use at least one of the Top 20 Power Foods to boost the foods from the Foundational Foods List. As you create your own meals and recipes (or explore the ones on my website), incorporate those power foods whenever you get the chance. But remember: This prescription is a combination of the micronutrients from the foods I selected *and* the style and timing of eating that repair the metabolic pathways being targeted right now.

GREEN APPLE WITH ALMOND BUTTER

Serves 1

> 1 Granny Smith apple, cored and sliced (see Note)
> 2 tablespoons almond butter

Dip the apple slices into the almond butter.

NOTE: Alternatively, core the apple and slice it in half horizontally (like an apple bagel), then smear the almond butter on one piece of the apple and top with the other slice of apple to make a sandwich.

QUINOA CRAB SALAD

Serves 2

> 1 cup quinoa
> 2 cups water
> 12 ounces lump crab meat
> 6 cups mâche salad mix
> 1 cup grated carrot
> 1 cup cherry tomatoes, halved
> 1 cup peeled, diced cucumber
> 3 tablespoons lemon juice
> Sea salt
> Freshly ground black pepper

In a medium saucepan, bring the quinoa and water to a boil over high heat. Cover, reduce the heat to low, and simmer until the quinoa is tender, about 15 minutes. Drain well; quinoa holds lots of water, so drain it thoroughly.

Place the quinoa in a large bowl and let cool. When room temperature, add the lettuce, vegetables, and lemon juice, and toss to combine. Season with salt and pepper to taste.

COD WITH SWEET MASH AND GREENS

Serves 2

> 2 medium sweet potatoes, washed
> 1½ teaspoons paprika
> Sea salt
> Freshly ground black pepper
> 2 6-ounce cod fillets

1 lemon, cut in quarters, seeds removed

2 cups vegetable broth

2 small shallots, sliced

4 garlic cloves, sliced

1 bunch collard greens, stems trimmed out, leaves chopped

$1/4$ teaspoon ground cinnamon

Preheat the oven to 400°F. Place the sweet potatoes on a baking sheet and bake for 45 to 60 minutes or until the potato is easily pierced with a fork.

Meanwhile, in a small mixing bowl, combine the paprika, $1/4$ teaspoon salt, and $1/4$ teaspoon black pepper. Season the cod with half the seasoning. Place the cod on a baking sheet. Squeeze half the lemon on the cod and bake for 12 to 15 minutes, until it flakes.

Meanwhile, in a sauté pan over high heat, combine the vegetable broth, shallots, garlic, collard greens, and the remaining seasoning mix. Cook for 10 minutes, or until all the liquid is absorbed. Season to taste with additional salt and pepper, if desired.

Peel the sweet potatoes, and use a potato masher or ricer to mash them. Add the cinnamon and a pinch of salt, if desired. Serve the cod fillets, mashed sweet potatoes, and collard greens on individual plates. Garnish each with a quarter of lemon.

RESTORE GI BALANCE: TOP THREE NON-FOOD STRATEGIES

Although food is your first line of defense as you prepare your gastrointestinal tract to best digest and assimilate nutrients, there are other effective actions you can take to facilitate this work and speed your progress. These are some of my favorite lifestyle strategies for improving digestive function:

- **Chew to the "Happy Birthday" song.** One of the easiest, cheapest, and most effective things you can do to improve your body's ability to fully digest your food is to chew your food thoroughly. A trick I like to tell my clients is to sing the "Happy Birthday" song while chewing each bite (not out loud of course—folks might think you're kooky, and your mouth is full!). Don't swallow until the song is over. This one habit can make a huge difference in how well you digest your food. Taking the time to chew stimulates more digestive juices than when you eat fast,

MORNING AND AFTERNOON SNACKS

Each of these snacks is a cooked vegetable, which you can prepare in any way you like—steamed, boiled, or even sautéed in an approved oil. You can puree your vegetables to make a soup and take them to work in a Thermos, or just cook them the night before (or use leftovers from dinner) and put them in a container to take to work. Cold roasted vegetables are yummy, or you can warm them in the microwave.

- Cooked Swiss chard
- Cooked Brussels sprouts
- Cooked asparagus
- Cooked spinach

EVENING SNACKS

As you can see, all these evening snacks are cooked fruit. You can bake these fruits or stew them in a little water until soft. Or, even grill or sauté them in a little approved oil.

- Cooked cherries
- Cooked plums
- Cooked pears
- Cooked apples

tossing the food down your gullet. Slow chewing also allows you to really mash up the food with saliva, so the digestion process starts before you swallow. My clients tell me it has practically cured everything from heartburn to constipation, and you may be much less likely to find undigested food in the toilet (gross). Don't underestimate the power of mastication!

- **Enjoy eating.** Your eating experience is crucial when you have GI dysfunction. Don't eat on the run or when you are upset or aggravated. Instead, sit down and enjoy your food. Notice your food. I don't care if you are also watching TV or listening to music; I hope you have time to enjoy great conversation during your meal. The point is to feel pleasure while eating. Pleasure hormones open metabolic pathways that allow you to digest your food more efficiently. So watch a comedy, or tell a joke, or laugh with your family or friends over dinner. Your GI tract will thank you.

- **Journal your meals and track your symptoms.** If you write down everything you eat and make note of how you felt after the meal and how you felt generally, GI-wise, you will start to recognize patterns. Journaling your meals and tracking your symptoms will give you solid information you can share with your doctor or natural health practitioner when you request lab tests or want additional advice on troubling symptoms.

BRIEFING YOUR DREAM TEAM

Your doctor may decide to run some lab tests to get to the bottom of your digestive issues, but there are a few tests I find helpful that doctors may not typically run. Ask for the following lab tests. Don't forget to write down your request, and include a list of your symptoms so the doctor can give the insurance company justification for ordering the tests. In my clinic, I use lab results the way some people use a scale to keep track of their weight. I use them to measure the success of the client's nutritional prescription. Running lab tests can also unveil important health issues that need to be addressed. If your lab results come back positive for some condition, talk to your doctor about possible courses of action. If this happens, you will also know that you are taking the right prescription.

- *Helicobacter pylori* **test:** This is a breath or stool test for the bacterium that causes inflammation of the stomach lining and that is also linked to stomach ulcers. A normal sample will not contain the *H. pylori* bacterium.

- **CDSA comprehensive digestive stool analysis:** This test detects the presence of yeast, parasites, and bacteria that contribute to chronic illness and neurological dysfunction.

- **Celiac disease test:** Celiac disease is an autoimmune disease, but particularly, the body attacks the small intestine, damaging your ability to digest and absorb nutrients. If you have this disease, you can never eat anything containing gluten, so it's important to know if you have the condition. Different doctors may decide to do different tests, and there are a number of tests that can be illuminating for celiac disease, so get your doctor's advice on which ones are right for you. The blood tests look at immunological reactions to the proteins in gluten, and are the first step in determining whether you might have celiac disease. If those tests come back negative, an intestinal biopsy can confirm the diagnosis. Note that you have to be eating gluten for test results to be accurate. If you have already quit eating gluten, you could get a false negative result. If you have celiac disease, you may want to begin with the autoimmune prescription (see Chapter 11).

- **Colorectal screening:** Colon cancer is an unusual but possible cause of digestive distress. Normally this involves a colonoscopy, but could also involve a blood test in those who cannot, for whatever reason, endure a colonoscopy.

- **C-reactive protein (CRP):** This test is a measure of inflammation. It is typically administered to determine heart disease risk, but it can also tell whether your digestive tract lining is likely to be chronically inflamed, as it measures system-wide inflammation.

- **Adult food allergy panel:** This test is controversial and there are some doctors who will tell you that the results are unreliable and unrelated to clinical symptoms. However, I like to run the IGM and IGG food allergy tests. These can give false negatives, but it is totally worth either avoiding or rotating foods in your diet that you react positively to.

SOMETHING TO CHEW ON

So many times, people say, "You are what you eat." Actually, you are what you have the ability to extract from your food. As you create your meal maps, and as you look to our community for additional recipes or you create your own, always keep in mind that the goal is to exploit the good in the food you eat, not to choose foods for what they lack.

This is a paradigm shift. Many people get so excited picking up a food and seeing it has only 100 calories or 1 gram of fat. We have been taught to get excited about "has less . . ." or "has fewer" or "has no . . ." foods, as in "has less sugar" or "has fewer calories" or "has no fat." Instead, what I want you to focus on is "has more," as in, "has more nutrient density." I want you to think about the *quality* of everything you put in your mouth. Do whatever you can to value and cherish that quality, whether it's chewing your food thoroughly or choosing the power foods. Be sure you make that paradigm shift. When you look down at your plate, ask: "What have you done for me lately? What can you do for me today?" Instead of thinking, "What don't you have?" think, "What *do* you have to enhance my health?"

CHAPTER 6

Fatigue, Low Energy, and Exhaustion

When your energy fluctuates—when you get fatigued, are exhausted, or feel bursts and sags of energy during the day, your body is whispering to you. Energy should work for you. You should have it when you need it throughout the day, and be able to sleep when the day is done. When neither is happening, your body is whispering that something is out of balance.

Energy issues are quite common, and although many people talk to their doctors about their fatigue and exhaustion, the tests a doctor runs might not reveal anything. Maybe you haven't manifested a disease, but your body just doesn't feel right. Many of my clients appear when a doctor told them everything looked fine—so why don't they feel well, they ask. Why can they barely drag themselves out of bed? Why are they falling asleep at their desks? Why is it so difficult just to get through the day? They've been told their symptoms are from stress or age or lack of sleep, and the recommendation is to "just get more sleep" or "lighten up on the stress" or even "just deal with it."

I have never been good with a "just deal with it" approach, and I also believe you can't tell someone to "just get more sleep" or "just lighten up" when the individual can't sleep or hasn't found a strategy that helps in de-stressing. So, in this chapter, we seek answers to why your energy levels are fluctuating. After all, you want to feel strong, good, and energetic, like a body should feel.

When your body is missing something, or is getting too much of something, or can't process or access something, it will downshift. Your energy level decreases, or becomes uneven, rising in spikes but then plunging. Eventually that fatigue and exhaustion can become chronic. The reason this happens is that tiny organelles inside most of your cells, called mitochondria, generate energy, called adenosine triphosphate (ATP). The ATP is the technical term, and so when I say "energy," that's what I mean. This energy is produced in the mitochondria using oxygen (which enters your body via your lungs), water, and the micronutrients in the foods you eat.

Without food, you wouldn't have any energy; and you can probably guess that the quality and substance of the foods you eat determine how well your mitochondria can produce the energy you need. If you aren't eating good, clean fuel, your energy output will suffer; and if any of the pathways for energy metabolism are blocked, your energy production will be reduced. Imagine there is a huge blizzard. You can't drive your car through the thick snow it leaves in your driveway. You have to shovel it out first to make a path. Similarly, to best optimize your internal energy production system, you need to fuel your mitochondria with targeted foods for the most efficient burning and clear out the metabolic pathways necessary to produce and utilize that energy.

THE SELF-DISCOVERY ZONE

What is it that your body is whispering to you? Are you dealing with fatigue, low energy, and exhaustion? There are subtle and sometimes not so subtle signs that you need a food prescription:

- Concentration or focus issues

- Dragging through the day, or fatigue all day long

- Energy slumps in the middle of the afternoon

- Exercise intolerance—your regular workout suddenly feels harder, or impossible, or you can't even seem to walk around the block very easily

- Falling asleep during the day, even at your desk

- Dry and weak hair

- Brittle nails

- Experiencing pain that moves around your body, like traveling bees

- Decreased sex drive—you just aren't ever in the mood anymore; it seems like too much effort

- Sexual dysfunction—you are having a hard time achieving an orgasm or erection

- Skin is crepe-like, hanging loosely with fine lines or wrinkles like wrinkled fabric

- Sleep issues—you have trouble falling or staying asleep at night

- Sleeping much more than usual and having a hard time waking up in the morning

- Decreased sports performance—you may be an athlete but discover you aren't running as quickly or playing as well as you used to

- Stimulant dependence—you are relying on stimulants such as coffee to get through a project or the day

- Have sugar and carbohydrate cravings

- Tired in the morning, even after you got enough sleep

- Weight gain when eating carbohydrates, and/or carbs and fats in combination

- Decreased work performance—you just don't seem to have the energy to give it your all

If this sounds like you, then your body is whispering for help. It has metabolically adapted to conserve its energy production and it is sending you all the right warning signals. Now is the time to repair the why—before your body has to raise its voice.

DEALING, NOT HEALING

One of the first things I ask my clients when they come into my office is, "If I had a magic wand and could make everything better, what would you want from your body?" Similarly, I want you to dream big. If you want the energy you had in your twenties, or the stamina to run a marathon, or to sleep deeply through the night and wake up truly refreshed, or just to be able to stand up during your child's entire soccer game, I want that for you, too. Whatever your goal, dream big and let's work toward it together. I always say to my clients, "We might not be able to do everything, but no ask is too big—because if you don't ask, we definitely can't achieve it."

If you visit a doctor complaining of low energy or sleep issues, chances are you won't be asked about your diet. Instead, your doctor will probably (or we hope) run some tests to see if you have any disorders that can cause low energy, such as low thyroid function, low iron/anemia, or low vitamin D. (At the end of this chapter I lay out strategic tools for partnering with your doctor and listening even more carefully, via diagnostics or lab tests, to what your body might be saying.)

If the tests your doctor chooses to run look normal, you may be diagnosed with a disorder that can't be specifically tested for but that is often diagnosed when nothing else is evident—something like chronic fatigue syndrome or fibromyalgia, if you also have pain. Or, you might be told to relax or exercise more or sleep more. You might get a prescription for sleeping pills. This is a reductionist approach to a complex metabolic disorder, and this is why so many people come to my clinics fully medicated, not fully well. What you need most is a nutrition prescription for balancing any or all of the metabolic pathways for energy metabolism.

WHAT SCIENCE SAYS IS TRUE

According to a study in the *Journal of Occupational and Environmental Medicine*, employees suffering from fatigue cost companies about $136.4 billion every year in lost productive time related to health issues, and fatigue was present in 37.9 percent of workers surveyed.* We are a tired bunch for sure, and there is a dollar cost, but what concerns me most is that people are missing out on the joy that an abundance of energy can bring.

_____

* J. A. Ricci et al., "Fatigue in the U.S. Workforce: Prevalence and Implications for Lost Productive Work Time," *Journal of Occupational and Environmental Medicine* 49, no. 1 (January 2007): 1–10.

TARGETED PATHWAYS FOR REPAIR

Energy is what gives us the capacity to run faster, jump higher, breathe deeper, create structure, and live our lives feeling healthy and strong, and to manifest the hormones that make the feeling of joy possible. Energy makes our hearts beat, keeps the blood flowing, fuels the secretion of hormones, grows hair, strengthens nails, and builds bone. Energy isn't just in the brain or the muscles. It is in every cell of our bodies, and if we don't have the energy currency to manufacture strong bones, muscles, and tissue, we eventually develop health issues, from weak nails and low bone density to reduced muscle tone and hormonal imbalances.

Energy is incredibly important for a successful and happy life. You can have all the money and possessions and fame in the world, but if you don't have any energy, you can't enjoy all those riches. When a client comes in and we choose to work toward restoring and reviving the person's energy levels, I focus on four energy pathways, and seek rebalance through food. Let's look at the four basic metabolic pathways that impact energy. You'll see soon how they all work together and why you want to target these for optimal energy output and metabolism.

ESSENTIAL ENERGY

This is a critical mode of energy production, which we use to live our everyday lives—it keeps the heart beating, muscles functioning, and brain working. I like to call it "Essential Energy" because it helps us do those things that are essential to daily life—walk to the water cooler and talk on the phone and prepare dinner and talk to our family and everything else we do all day long. So, you have to do something to get this kind of energy—you have to eat. This energy comes from the mitochondria using oxygen to burn sugar that comes from carbohydrate-rich foods. This is the easiest and quickest way for the body to create energy.

If you think of the total possible energy production in your body being worth $100, Essential Energy would be worth about $30, or 30 percent of your ideal energy pool for the day. So, if you can eat carbs, break them down into sugar, and convert that sugar into energy, you're more than a third of the way there. For those having issues with energy metabolism, however, that's hard to do. And remember: You have to eat for this process to work. If you don't, your body will cannibalize the muscle and the liver, because those places are where the body stores sugar.

CREATED ENERGY

This is the energy boost we get from exercise and other kinds of physical exertion. Because exercise takes more energy than everyday living, it triggers the body to upregulate, or speed up its energy consumption; we burn fuel at an increased rate in the mitochondria, and that triggers the production of more energy. This kind of energy works differently from essential energy, though. When we exercise, we use up the oxygen in our tissues. For Essential Energy, we need oxygen to burn sugar. But because during exercise the oxygen is depleted, the body opens up a new pathway to burn sugar and create more energy. Smart body!

This newly opened channel is called the "lactic acid pathway." This creates a burst of extra energy, and it's great for short-term intense exercise, such as sprints or rapid reps or HIIT (high intensity interval training) programs. It doesn't last very long, though. It is not sustainable, but it can be enhanced by conditioning. And get this—it can be increased by what you eat before you exercise. Although it's good energy, in the scheme of total energy production it only nets you about $5 of that $100, or 5 percent of your daily energy desire. It also helps both Essential Energy and Metabolic Energy (see next section) work better, though, so it has those added benefits—consider it interest in the bank. There are endless health benefits to exercise, but I do not believe increasing exercise alone can repair fatigue, low energy, and exhaustion—and yet, so many of my tapped-out clients are told to "just work out more."

METABOLIC ENERGY

This is the very best kind of energy—it is slow, steady, rich, and even. It makes us feel physically strong, and when this metabolic pathway is flowing, it quenches the body's thirst for energy abundantly. It is like a river of water, compared to a bottle. We feel limitless, not slightly stimulated. It's the difference between feeling wound up and feeling fired up. Metabolic energy can make you feel steady and well fueled all day long. And it comes from burning fat for fuel instead of sugar.

When the mitochondria burn fat to produce ATP, the result is cleaner (meaning there are fewer by-products of energy metabolism, like free radicals, which can cause wrinkles and advanced aging and inflammation) than when it burns sugar. It is the most metabolically efficient form of energy metabolism. If you have a lot of fat to burn, both on your body and from your diet of healthy fats, you can think of that as tons of potential energy. If you have extra pockets of fat where you don't want them, however, this means your fat-burning pathways may not be working as well as they should. These pockets are your piggy bank, your reserve; if you can access them, you can burn that fat and feel great! But to get the fat burning started, you have to eat. It takes enzymes and bile salt. (It's E + M = H again.) Because this kind of energy produces so much more ATP, it nets you a cool $60, or more than half your bankroll.

CRISIS ENERGY

This last form of energy is the most adjustable and the most influenced by environment, food, lifestyle, and stress levels. It's crisis fuel. We shouldn't need much of it on a daily basis, but if we are lacking or lagging in essential, created, or metabolic energy (or all three), the Crisis Energy picks up the slack.

This can happen for many reasons, such as when you aren't metabolizing sugar and fat sufficiently, when you aren't able to move enough, or when you are under stress. Stress of any kind can generate Crisis Energy—you might be stressed from lack of sleep, lack of food, lack of joy, physical trauma, or even emotional trauma. Even good stress can generate Crisis Energy; think of a new job, a new home, a new spouse, or a new baby.

Crisis Energy is generated from the release of glucocorticoids like cortisol, epinephrine, and norepinephrine—what are often called the "stress hormones." This spurs what I refer to as a "futile energy cycle," whereby your body starts burning anything and everything it can for energy in order to have enough energy to manage the crisis it feels it is experiencing, whether that consumption is muscle, bone, hair, skin, or teeth.

Many people are living on Crisis Energy production. When they depend on this, it creates a cascade of disruption in metabolic pathways correlated with everything from depression to autoimmune disorders to cancers. In a healthy human, Crisis Energy should only be worth about $5, or 5 percent of your energy, but unfortunately, so many people suffer from chronic stress that they are operating on 75 percent or more Crisis Energy. This exhausts the body, especially the adrenal glands and everything downstream of them.

REMOVE, REPAIR, AND RESTORE

The goal is to develop a nutrition prescription that supports your body's ability to metabolize sugar, carbs (Essential Energy), and fat (Metabolic Energy), and that maximizes your exercise efforts (Created Energy) and lowers the need to access energy via the stress hormones (Crisis Energy). You want to reestablish a healthier balance of energy. To do this, you will:

1. Remove blockages to sugar and fat metabolism.

2. Repair mitochondrial function with targeted power foods.

3. Restore healthy mechanisms for burning sugar and fat for fuel.

GUIDELINES FOR YOUR ENERGY REPAIR RX

Here's what you need to know about eating for energy:

- You will be taking this prescription five times a day (in other words, you will be eating five times a day). You will also split each week into two parts, eating one way for four consecutive days and then another way for three consecutive days. Then you will repeat this eating pattern.

- Typically my clients stay on this program for a minimum of three months, or at least one month for every year they have heard any or all energy-related whispers. Because each of the healthy food groups is represented in this prescription, many people continue to eat this way permanently; you don't have to stop as long as it is working for you. But don't forget to revisit the Self-Discovery Zone in this chapter, so you keep listening to the whispers and notice when they stop.

- If you are allergic, don't like, or have religious or ethical objections to any of the foods on the list, simply avoid those and replace them with different foods in the same category on the Top 20 Power Foods for Energy Repair list. For example, you can exchange asparagus for spinach or cantaloupe for raspberries.

- Tell your doctor that you are using a food prescription to work on your energy issues. This is a tough one for you to get support from most doctors, but what you can say is, "I have noticed a change in my health, and because it's a change, I am concerned; and it is not a change I am willing to go forward with." You can also be more specific; for instance, you might add, "I used to be able to run five miles, and now I can only do two." Or, "I typically only need eight hours of sleep, and I've been sleeping for ten to twelve hours or I can't function, and this alarms me." This tells your doctor that you want help, and your doctor may then be more willing to run the lab tests you request (which you can find toward the end of this chapter). Remember to drink half your body weight in ounces of spring water every day, with a maximum of 100 ounces per day.

EAT YOUR MEDICINE: YOUR ENERGY REPAIR RX

Opposite are the power foods to focus on as you choose how to fill in your meal maps.

As for your meal maps, this prescription has a two-part meal map. The first part you follow for the first four days of each week, or days 1–4, and the second part you follow for the last three days of the week, or days 5–7. Follow this pattern each week for three months, unless your energy dip is very recent (in which case you can default to the rule of thumb for eating this way for one month for every year you have been feeling these whispers). Do not deviate from the order and food categories as they are laid out here, but you can change the specific foods selected from each category. Just be sure that, for example, the first four days include a high-glycemic fruit and a healthy fat for snack. That rule is nonnegotiable.

My strategy in the first four days of this meal map is to stimulate energy production by providing the body with both natural sugar from fruit (but not grain) and healthy fat for better fat metabolism, and removing the complex carbs in the form of grain, while using strategically placed vegetables to stimulate the enzymes that stabilize the rate of sugar delivery from the fruit.

Emphasize these power foods, incorporating them into your meals whenever possible:

Asparagus

Brussels sprouts

Cantaloupe

Cauliflower

Celery

Chiles

Coconut oil

Cucumbers

Eggs

Fish—wild-caught, except tilapia, grouper, or catfish

Ginger, fresh or ground

Grapefruit

Lemons

Lentils

Meats—all lean types

Nuts, raw

Oatmeal

Quinoa

Raspberries

Spinach

MEAL MAP FOR ENERGY REPAIR, DAYS 1–4

BREAKFAST	SNACK	LUNCH	SNACK	DINNER
Protein Healthy Fat	Fruit (high G.I.) Healthy Fat	Protein Fruit (high G.I.) Vegetable	Fruit (high G.I.) Healthy Fat	Protein Fruit (high G.I.) Vegetable

This plan stimulates the metabolism of digested fats in the first part of the week. During the second half of the week, or the last three days of the week, the strategy is to pull the dietary fats out, so the body begins to catabolize, or break down, the stored fat for energy, stimulating the natural pathway of

Metabolic Energy. This is a big job, which is why you need to cycle through the week in the prescribed way, fluctuating between times of rest and restoration, and then of rebuilding and stimulating.

MEAL MAP FOR ENERGY REPAIR, DAYS 5–7

BREAKFAST	SNACK	LUNCH	SNACK	DINNER
Complex Carb Vegetable Fruit (low G.I.)	Complex Carb Vegetable	Protein Vegetable Fruit (low G.I.)	Complex Carb Vegetable	Protein Vegetable

A DAY IN THE LIFE OF ENERGY REPAIR

Let's look at a sample day for each of the two parts of the week and see how you might use the Foundational Foods List punctuated with the targeted energy power foods to create your own meal plan. Day 1 shows how you might eat during the first part of the 4/3 split, and day 5 shows how you might choose to eat during the second part. Following each sample meal map are some recipes to get you started. The meal items in boldface indicate the recipes included here.

SAMPLE DAY FOR ENERGY REPAIR, DAYS 1–4

BREAKFAST	SNACK	LUNCH	SNACK	DINNER
Baked Avocado with Egg	Mango slices with pistachios	**Cantaloupe Salad**	Pear and almond milk	**Pineapple Stir-fry**

RECIPES

Notice that I incorporated choices from the Top 20 Power Foods list into these recipes so as to boost the power of the prescription. As you get more comfortable with eating this way and explore more recipe ideas, remember to add power foods whenever you can, but also remember that the timing and types of food for each meal are an equally important part of this prescription.

BAKED AVOCADO WITH EGG

Serves 2

  1 medium avocado
  2 large eggs
  2 teaspoons lemon juice
  Sea salt
  Freshly ground black pepper
  1 tablespoon thinly sliced green onion (white parts)

Preheat the oven to 425°F.

Slice the avocado in half, and take out the pit. Scoop out a little bit of flesh from each half's center—just enough so an egg will fit snugly in the cavity (and don't waste it—eat the part you scoop out!). Place the avocado halves in a small baking dish; do your best to make sure they fit tightly so they don't tip over. Crack an egg into each avocado half, pouring the yolk in first and then letting the white fill in the space. Place in the oven and bake for 15 to 20 minutes. (The cooking time varies depending on the size of your avocado; just make sure the white is set.)

Remove the avocado from the oven, then drizzle each avocado half with lime juice and season to taste with salt and pepper. Sprinkle the tops with green onion and serve.

CANTALOUPE SALAD

Serves 2

  2 cups cubed cantaloupe (cut into ¾- to 1-inch cubes)
  8 ounces prosciutto, black forest ham, or smoked ham (nitrate free only)
  3 tablespoons lime juice
  3 tablespoons chopped fresh mint
  2 teaspoons grated lime zest
  1 teaspoon grated fresh ginger
  Sea salt

Place the cantaloupe in a large bowl. Dice the prosciutto or ham and add it to the bowl. Sprinkle on the lime juice, mint, and lime zest; toss to blend. Mix in the ginger, then sprinkle to taste with salt. Refrigerate the salad until ready to serve, stirring occasionally.

PINEAPPLE STIR-FRY

Serves 4

$^1/_2$ cup chicken or vegetable broth

$^1/_4$ cup tamari

$^1/_2$ tablespoon minced fresh ginger

1 cup cubed fresh pineapple (in $^1/_2$-inch pieces)

1 large whole boneless, skinless chicken breast (get a large breast weighing about 1 pound—if packaged in halves, use 2), cut into $^1/_2$-inch cubes

$^1/_2$ cup sliced onion

1 cup shredded carrots

$^1/_2$ cup thinly sliced celery

1 cup sugar-snap peas, ends trimmed

1 small red bell pepper, cored, seeded, and sliced

2 lemons, halved and seeded

2 tablespoons thinly sliced green onion, white and green parts

Sea salt

Freshly ground black pepper

In a medium saucepan over high heat, combine the broth, tamari, ginger, and pineapple. Bring to a boil and reduce the heat to medium. Cook for 10 minutes, or until the liquid has reduced by about half.

In a sauté pan or wok over high heat, place 3 tablespoons of the pineapple sauce and add the chicken. Cook for 5 to 6 minutes. Remove from the heat and transfer to a plate.

Place the pan back over high heat. Add the onion, carrots, celery, sugar-snap peas, red pepper, and remaining sauce. Squeeze 2 of the lemon halves into the mixture and then toss in the lemon halves themselves. Cook until the vegetables are tender, 3 to 4 minutes. Remove from the heat, then remove and discard the lemon halves.

Add the chicken and toss to combine. Place the stir-fry on individual plates and garnish with the green onion and remaining lemon halves, cutting each half in half again. Season with $^1/_2$ teaspoon salt and $^1/_4$ teaspoon pepper, or to taste.

- Pineapple cubes tossed in shredded coconut, cherries, and raw almonds
- Apple slices with cashew butter
- Orange slices tossed with cinnamon and shredded coconut
- Peach slices and walnuts

SAMPLE DAY FOR ENERGY REPAIR, DAYS 5-7

BREAKFAST	SNACK	LUNCH	SNACK	DINNER
Spinach Mushroom Wrap	Brown rice crackers and celery sticks	**Hawaiian Chicken Soup**	Spelt pretzels and raw cauliflower and broccoli florets	**Salmon in Foil**

RECIPES

SPINACH MUSHROOM WRAP

Serves 4

10 ounces white, crimini, or baby bella mushrooms, cleaned and sliced

10 ounces fresh baby spinach

1 cup water

2 Roma (plum) tomatoes, chopped

1/4 cup chopped onion

1 tablespoon minced garlic

2 tablespoons chopped fresh parsley

1 tablespoon chopped fresh cilantro

Sea salt

Freshly ground black pepper

4 sprouted-grain or spelt tortillas

1 cup alfalfa sprouts

Salsa of choice (optional)

Combine the mushrooms, half the spinach, and the water in a large sauté pan over high heat. Cook for 2 to 3 minutes, or until the mushrooms have softened and the spinach has wilted. Add the tomatoes, onion, garlic, parsley, and cilantro;

cook for 1 minute. Add the remaining spinach, season to taste with salt and pepper, and cook until the added spinach has wilted.

Meanwhile, warm the tortillas in a pan over low heat.

Spoon some of the spinach mixture on the tortillas. Top each with ¼ cup alfalfa sprouts. Add salsa, if desired. Tuck the sides of the tortillas into the center and roll up to create the wraps.

HAWAIIAN CHICKEN SOUP

Serves 4 (serving size: 2 cups)

- 3 cups diced fresh pineapple
- 3 cups water
- 1 14.5-ounce can low-sodium chicken broth
- 1-inch piece of fresh ginger, sliced
- 2 garlic cloves, smashed
- 1 tablespoon coconut aminos
- Zest of 2 lemons
- 1 cup trimmed clamshell mushrooms, or use thinly sliced oyster or shiitake mushrooms
- 1 pound boneless, skinless chicken thighs, cubed
- ½ serrano chile
- 1 teaspoon sea salt
- Freshly ground black pepper
- 1 green onion, thinly sliced

Blend 1 cup of the pineapple with the water in a blender until smooth, about 1 minute. Strain into a 4-quart pot. Add the broth, ginger, garlic, coconut aminos, and lemon zest. Simmer over medium heat, covered, until the flavors have melded, 10 to 15 minutes. Strain and discard the solids.

Place the broth mixture back into the pot and add the remaining 2 cups pineapple, the mushrooms, chicken, and chile. Cook over medium heat until the chicken is firm, about 10 minutes. Add the salt and season to taste with pepper. Serve in bowls garnished with the green onion.

SALMON IN FOIL

Serves 2

> 2 6-ounce wild-caught salmon fillets
> Sea salt
> Freshly ground black pepper
> 1½ tablespoons whole-grain mustard
> 1 tablespoon minced fresh tarragon
> 2 cups chopped trimmed asparagus
> 2 lemons, each cut into 4 slices

Preheat the oven to 425°F.

Season the salmon with ½ teaspoon salt and ¼ teaspoon pepper. In a mixing bowl, blend the mustard and tarragon. Spread the mixture on top of the salmon.

Cut two pieces of foil long enough to encase each salmon fillet when folded over the center and up on the ends. Position the foil pieces on a large baking sheet and place 1 cup asparagus in the center of each foil, season with a little salt and pepper, and place 2 lemon slices on top. Put the salmon fillets on top of the asparagus, skin side down. Place 2 more lemon slices on top of each salmon fillet. Fold the edges of the foil up over the salmon and crimp to seal. Fold the edges together on both ends to create two airtight packages.

Bake the salmon packets for 15 to 20 minutes, or until just cooked through but still moist. Transfer the packets to individual plates. Slip open the tops of the packets carefully, releasing some steam, and spoon any accumulated juices over the fish.

SNACK IDEAS FOR ENERGY REPAIR, DAYS 5–7

- Brown rice crackers and bell pepper slices
- Spelt tortilla rolled up with mixed salad veggies (can add a little olive oil and apple cider vinegar or citrus juice, if desired)
- Sprouted-grain toast and jícama sticks
- Leftover brown or wild rice tossed with chopped fresh kale or romaine lettuce and shredded carrots
- Small spinach salad with sprouted-grain croutons (you can use a little oil and citrus juice on top, if desired)

RESTORE ENERGY BALANCE: TOP THREE NON-FOOD STRATEGIES

In addition to your food prescription, there are some powerful strategies with which you can infuse your body with energy and balance your energy production and metabolism pathways. Add one, two, or all three of these to your life and feel the energy come flooding back in.

EXERCISE FOR MORE ENERGY

Doctors and other health-care professionals often recommend increasing exercise as a remedy for energy issues, but the last thing you want to do when your energy is low is further tax your body with strenuous exercise. Yet, exercise can be a valuable tool in restoring energy. You just have to take it easy. Here are some guidelines:

1. Keep your heart rate on the low side. Exercising at a slower pace is more likely to stimulate the burning of fat than will the burning of glycogen in your muscles and organs that happen with vigorous exercise, so dial it back. The best way to measure this is by tracking your heart rate during exercise. Keep your heart rate between 125 and 135 beats per minute throughout the workout. A simple heart monitor or fitness tracker that measures heart rate will help you do this. Some gym machines also do this for you.

   You can also track your oxygen saturation with a pulse oximeter. This equipment is a little harder to come by, but their price is coming down as they get more popular. I find it very useful because it tracks how much oxygen I am burning. Remember that Essential Energy requires oxygen to burn sugar, so one important goal for energy restoration is to not burn through too much oxygen during exercise—not until you have restored healthy energy metabolism. Measure your resting oxygen saturation, and then during exercise, don't let it drop more than two or three points. If it drops more than that, stop exercising, take a few moments to breathe to restore oxygen, then start again. Five points is the absolute maximum you should push it to if you are exercising for energy restoration.

2. Exercise early in the day, preferably before 2:00 p.m., rather than in the late afternoon or evening. Earlier in the day, your adrenal output tends to function better; later in the day, it produces the hormones that trigger Crisis Energy.

3. Eat either a high G.I. fruit and a healthy fat (if you are in the first four days of the week) or a complex carb and veggie (if you are in the last three days of the week) thirty minutes before your workout. This provides your body with adequate amounts of food-based sugars to fuel the muscles, so your body will use those for fuel rather than scavenging muscle tissue.

SLEEP FOR MORE ENERGY

How, when, and under what conditions you sleep can make a real difference in how well your body manages energy production and metabolism. These strategies will help make your sleep as powerful and rejuvenating as possible:

1. Nix the electronic stimulation in your sleep environment. Whenever possible, get rid of computers, alarm clocks, televisions, and cell phones in the room where you sleep. Electronics are stimulating to the body and can prevent you from obtaining deep sleep.

2. Keep your sleep environment dark. The pineal gland, right behind your eyes, responds well to darkness. This is the gland that produces melatonin, which helps regulate your sleep cycles. Eyelids are somewhat translucent, so even with the eyes closed, a lighted environment will negatively influence the pineal gland. Not only do televisions and lights interfere with sleep but so does the light from windows. Consider blackout shades.

3. Get eight hours of sleep. So you didn't clean the whole house yet? You still haven't watched your favorite show? When you are working to repair low energy, fatigue, and exhaustion, those things can wait. You need a minimum of eight hours of sleep per night when you are restocking your energy piggy bank. If this is impossible (or even if it's possible but you still feel fatigued) a fifteen- to forty-five-minute nap in the afternoon can also be very restorative. Remember, you are trying to

heal, not just deal. Even if you can only take a nap during the first two weeks of this program, you will make a big difference in your healing process. Ideally, you'll do it for the entire three months, because every time you take a nap, it's like putting money into that bank.

PASSIVE STRESS REDUCTION

There are many stress-reduction techniques out there, but some take more energy and physical or mental engagement than others. Although I'm a fan of things like yoga and meditation, they can be stressful for some people. They take effort, concentration, and commitment, and they represent one more thing to put on the schedule that can make you feel stressed. Instead, right now, as you are working to restore energy, focus on passive stress-reduction techniques—things that happen to you rather than things you have to do. If you can just show up and lie on a table and have somebody rub your back, or do other things to make you feel better, then what's to stress about? Any of the following examples are good if you have access to professionals who employ them (take their advice on how to proceed with them, as these therapies are highly individual):

- Massage

- Essential oils

- Homeopathy

- Acupuncture

These passive activities will help shift your body's ability to rebalance your energy pathways. Remember that vigorous exercise, yoga, meditation, alternate nostril breathing, and many of the other stress-management techniques that are so popular now are great for many objectives, but for energy restoration, keep it passive. If all you can do each week is get a massage, that's awesome. If a professional is too pricey, enlist a loved one. Agree to take turns. Just being touched is therapeutic.

BRIEFING YOUR DREAM TEAM

If you're not feeling like yourself, don't take that feeling lightly. Along with your annual physical and baseline tests your doctor may recommend, there are a few other tests that are helpful. These aren't anything unusual, but your doctor may not order them unless you ask for them, as he or she might not think your energy downturn is necessarily lab worthy. However, the results of these tests can be illuminating. You will be looking for things that might traditionally be missed in other lab tests—things that are out of balance from a chemical perspective. But don't discount your symptoms even if your labs are normal; sometimes the body can be significantly out of balance and that won't necessarily show up in the blood chemistry. You just want to rule out anything that may need additional support, and have the objective tools to measure your success.

- **Ferritin level:** Ferritin is a protein made by the liver that binds to iron. It is essential for carrying and delivering iron and oxygen from the bloodstream into the cells and is required to convert carbs, sugars, and fats into energy. Oftentimes, a person may not appear anemic when iron levels are measured, but there may be a ferritin issue, making it difficult for the body to deliver iron and oxygen. Low ferritin levels are often associated with fatigue; ask for a ferritin level test even if you have normal iron and hemoglobin numbers.

- **CK level:** CK, or creatine kinase, is found in the blood specifically when muscle tissue is being broken down. Normal levels mean the body isn't breaking down muscle very much. If the level is high, this could be an indication that the body is using the metabolic pathways for breaking down muscle for energy. This can happen when you aren't well hydrated; also, some individuals are prone to scavenging muscle instead of fat.

- **Testosterone level:** This is an important test for both men and women when energy is an issue. If it's low, apart from any libido issues, this can be a sign that an individual is not getting restorative sleep. If you are sleeping eight hours but waking up feeling like you haven't slept at all, your sleep is probably not restoring you and you are probably not producing enough testosterone. If you have low testosterone, you might benefit from a melatonin supplement in addition to the other sleep advice given in this chapter. I can't tell you how many clients come in who have sleep apnea and low T. When we repair the sleep apnea, the testosterone levels go through the roof! This is why I am not generally in favor of simply supplementing with testosterone, which many health-care professionals recommend. It's not that I'm diametrically opposed to hormone replacement therapy, but I believe that we should optimize the body before considering that treatment. I would rather get to the bottom of why a client's body isn't producing enough testosterone, or why it isn't being used, and fix that. Then, with a little help scrubbing the receptor sites and restoring the pathways with the right micronutrients from food, the body is more likely to fix the hormone levels itself. (I talk more about testosterone and other reproductive hormones in Chapter 7.)

SOMETHING TO CHEW ON

The biggest paradigm shift I see with my clients when we are working on this prescription is to understand the value of rest for restoration. So much of the repair process happens when the body sleeps. As you start to have more energy, don't be quick to burn that newly created resource. When you've had enough rest that you start to have a little bit of extra energy, that's when you should lie down, so that the energy can do the work for complete repair.

When I have clients coming out of extreme energy slumps, I always notice that as their energy grows, so do their to-do lists. Oh no, no, my friend! You are doing this so you can repair the fragile metabolic pathways that got you into this state. Time resting is never time wasted. Every day that you begin to feel more energy, have a designated hour of afternoon rest.

Be cognizant about where that energy is going. Understand that it is not a matter of "overdoing it," but in allowing that precious energy to regenerate healthy tissue—your skin, hair, nails, bone, muscles, and organs. There will be more stressors coming down the pike—chemical, physical, emotional, or whatever. The more vital energy you can create now, coursing through your functional pathways, the better your body will be able to adapt to changes in its environment.

PART THREE

Your Body Is Talking

CHAPTER 7

PMS, Perimenopause, Menopause, and "Manopause"

It's kind of a crazy undertaking—attacking all the hormonal symptoms in one chapter, right? Well, remember, we aren't chasing symptoms. We are getting at the heart of the message your body is sending to you and going to the essence or root cause—the why. We are focusing on the major metabolic pathways that support all hormonal function or dysfunction. The hormones behave like a complex, intertwined balancing act. When an imbalance occurs, a variety of symptoms can appear, from weight gain, to hair loss, to pain; these symptoms can set the stage for major chronic diseases. When your body starts talking hormonal imbalance, it's a message you need to hear.

There are many hormones in the body, but in this chapter we shine the spotlight on what we call the "sex hormones." These hormones have a major influence on many systems and functions in the body, and when those pathways are disrupted, the body lets us know. For instance, when your body is taking on stubborn fat that doesn't want to budge and you're suffering from mood swings and seemingly random pain, you may have a hormonal imbalance. Hormones are extremely powerful; they can influence many more systems downstream, so nipping imbalances in the bud with a nutritional prescription *now* can not only make your PMS milder and cool your hot flashes but can make you feel more like yourself all month long (guys, too!). The symptoms can come via other pathways in the body, but when they happen because of hormones, there is a specific nutritional prescription just for you.

THE SELF-DISCOVERY ZONE

If your hormones are out of balance, you may be manufacturing, detoxifying, recycling, or metabolizing too little or too much of a given class of hormones, such as estrogen, progesterone, or testosterone (or a combination of any of these). Your stress hormones, or the hormones that regulate the blood sugar, can also influence or inhibit the sex hormones. When this happens, many other systems are affected down the line, so it is important to address your body's talk before it is forced to scream. Here are some specific things that are likely to start happening in your body when hormones are out of balance:

- Breasts are tender or painful, and can change shape or density, either cyclically or change and stay that way.

- Less energy or fatigue

- Foggy brain

- Forgetfulness

- Hot flashes

- Insomnia or other sleep issues

- Men—not having a morning erection

- Mood swings, quickly changing from elation to irritation or anger

- Night sweats

- Periods that become heavier or form large clots

- Periods that become irregular, either more often or less often

- PMS symptoms getting worse—more bloating, cramps, irritability, and mood swings

- Sex drive declines or disappears

- Urine leakage when sneezing, coughing, or laughing

- Vaginal dryness that is uncomfortable or interferes with sexual activity

- Weepiness or excessive emotion

- Rapid and sudden weight gain

If you have many of these symptoms, your body is talking to you, saying that something is out of balance. Even if your basic blood chemistry looks stable and is within normal ranges, if your body is experiencing these symptoms you want to pay attention. It might mean your hormonal system isn't working correctly, which is causing trouble that you are metabolically adapting to. Let's repair the situation so the problem doesn't advance to something chronic and more difficult to resolve.

DEALING, NOT HEALING

I do not believe you have to "muscle through" menopause or struggle with a low libido. Until you hit 100 years old, I will not accept the excuse that hormonal discomfort is just "what you get" when you age. Hormones change all the time, but that doesn't mean you should settle for less than feeling good, even in the face of hormonal fluctuations.

If you don't tend to your hormones, the imbalances will worsen; they won't simply go away. You don't have to accept being out of control of your body or live with a softening waistline. Hormone imbalances are not something to "just deal with." Because hormones regulate and activate many other metabolic pathways, such as ones that cause cancer, heart disease, and possibly even Alzheimer's, we need to take seriously these messages our bodies are sending us and eat in a way to rebalance the metabolic pathways.

Wouldn't it be awesome if your PMS could just disappear? If you could be over and done with menopause without pain and discomfort? If you could enjoy the energy, vigor, and sex drive you get with normal testosterone levels? You have the right to want those things, and they are within your reach.

If you have a hormone imbalance, which your doctor will diagnose if your lab tests show an abnormal excess or deficiency of sex hormones, the typical treatments involve medication: birth control pills, hormone replacement therapy, progesterone patches or IUDs, testosterone supplements, even antidepressants. Food is unlikely to enter the discussion, even though we know that food has a profound effect on hormone balance and the ability of the body to both manufacture and metabolize the hormones that control so many major metabolic processes in the body.

People who carry a lot of fat stores tend to have more circulating hormones in their bloodstream than people who have less fat, and they are not actively utilizing, metabolizing, or detoxifying these hormones. This is because fat cells can produce their own hormones. This can lead to imbalanced levels and more uncomfortable PMS and premenopausal symptoms, as well as an increased risk for hormone-receptor–positive breast cancer. A 2012 study showed that this situation can be remedied, however.* The study divided 439 overweight or obese postmenopausal women who were generally sedentary into four groups. One group was given a healthy diet and met regularly with a dietitian. Another group was put on a moderate to vigorous exercise plan. The third group was given the diet plus exercise. And the fourth group was given no particular instruction (the control group). The researchers tracked hormone levels in all these women, and the results in the diet-only and diet-and-exercise groups showed significant decreases in estrone and estradiol (both forms of estrogen) and testosterone, as well as significant increases in sex hormone–binding globulin (SHBG), which binds to hormones and carries them out of the body. (This is what you want if your fat cells are overproducing hormones.) The exercise-only group showed some improvement in all these factors, but much less than the diet-only group. The diet-plus-exercise group was the clear winner, lowering hormones and increasing SHBG hormone levels the most.

---

* K. L. Campbell et al., "Reduced-Calorie Dietary Weight Loss, Exercise, and Sex Hormones in Postmenopausal Women: Randomized Controlled Trial," *Journal of Clinical Oncology* 30, no. 10 (July 1, 2012): 2314–26.

TARGETED PATHWAYS FOR REPAIR

Hormones trigger metabolic activity in so many ways that any hormonal imbalance will, if left uncorrected, eventually result in a host of issues, from weight gain to chronic disease. For your hormone nutritional prescription, we will:

1. STIMULATE THE PATHWAYS THAT METABOLIZE STORED FAT IN THE BODY.

Stored fat in the body disrupts the sex hormone balance, as well as blood sugar regulation and immune function. We want your body to scavenge the stored fat because this fat is creating excess hormones. Normally, the sex glands—the ovaries and testes—as well as some of the other glands in your body produce or trigger the production of estrogen. However, if you have extra body fat, compensatory hormones are also being created by your fat cells. The more fat you have, the more hormones will be produced, and they may not be able to be used, creating excessive amounts in the blood, typically of estrogen (even in men). This can interfere with weight, mood, behavior, and many aspects of metabolic function.

2. SUPPORT PREGNENOLONE (MASTER HORMONE) PRODUCTION.

The body converts cholesterol molecules into a master hormone called pregnenolone, which is a precursor to all the other hormones. For pregnenolone to do its work, however, we must first effectively metabolize cholesterol, so it can then convert pregnenolone into estrogen, progesterone, and testosterone—all the sex hormones, as well as the blood sugar regulating hormones, stress hormones, and immune-regulating hormones. When there is a problem with the manufacture of hormones from cholesterol, cholesterol metabolism may be impaired. Cholesterol is essential for the creation of hormones, and when you can't metabolize cholesterol, you are more likely to develop a hormonal deficiency (often of progesterone or testosterone, but also of estrogen).

3. IMPROVE VITAMIN D MANUFACTURE, STORAGE, OR METABOLISM.

Vitamin D is a crucial component of hormone function and creation, so when there is a problem with the body's ability to manufacture, store, and/or metabolize vitamin D, there may be hormonal deficiency or imbalance. We need to effectively wash the receptor sites so the hormones can be received by the appropriate cells, reigniting the body's demand for hormone production. This sounds complex, and the way I like to describe it to my clients is this: If I were to ask if you have groceries in your refrigerator—if we opened your fridge and it was full of food—you wouldn't feel the need to go to the grocery store. Even if the food were expired, rotten, not what you wanted to eat, or unhealthy, your first instinct would be to see the fridge as full. But when we clean out the fridge and you get rid of all the stuff that is rotten or moldy or past its expiration date, you realize you have a demand for groceries. Hey, the fridge is empty!

So, let's go shopping. With hormones, the receptor sites can get gummed

MANOPAUSE: FACT OR FICTION?

Although medical hormonal discussions are more commonly centered on women and their monthly fluctuations, men are just as subject to hormonal imbalances, which some people call "manopause." This is a silly name for a serious condition—that happens when the male body begins to adapt dysfunctionally by creating imbalances in hormone production and metabolism. Clinically, I see this starting to happen with men beginning as early as the late thirties. Symptoms include loss of muscle mass, thickening in the hips, softer and fattier pectoral muscles, pooling serum cholesterol, low energy, changes in libido, premature ejaculation and other performance issues, thinning of hair on the head and body, fatigue, lack of inspiration and drive, memory and cognition issues, and that six-pack turning into a pony keg.

A man's ability to convert hormones is efficient, and those efficient metabolic conversion pathways are quick to back-convert testosterone into estrogen as men age. Men are also subject to inflammatory imbalances like elevated homocysteine and C-reactive protein. Doctors are often focused on the cardiovascular implications of these test results, and they can raise a man's heart disease risk. But these changes are also a major indication of dysfunctional hormone conversion.

Men also have cycles, but they tend to be seasonal rather than monthly. There are many theories about why this is true, including the idea that early man was outside more and more subject to the changing seasons while hunting. I'm not sure I believe that, but I have witnessed, clinically, that these seasonal shifts happen in my male clients.

up, tricking the body into thinking it has enough of a hormone when it is actually deficient, the hormone metabolites are incomplete, or the hormones are in dysfunctional forms and can't be utilized. The fridge looks full, but it isn't. Thinking it is, the body starts to lower hormone production. When you wash receptor sites and clean out all the junk, it reestablishes demand for your body's natural production, and then you can reestablish a healthy homeostasis with adequate hormone production. Vitamin D is important in this process because of its ability to be manufactured in and stored by the body. That is why I always say that when I see a low serum vitamin D result in my clients' lab tests, I am beyond suspicious that a hormone imbalance is causing it. We don't want to just supplement. We want to understand the why.

4. FEED THE GLANDS RESPONSIBLE FOR HORMONE SECRETION.

It is so common in my practice to see clients whose adrenal glands, ovaries, testes, pituitary, and thyroid aren't being nurtured appropriately. The body begins to depend on fat cells to make up for this lack of hormone production. So, we have to feed the glands that produce the appropriate hormone balance most efficiently and productively.

REMOVE, REPAIR, AND RESTORE

Our objective with this prescription is to help your body manufacture and utilize hormones in the most efficient way possible. Sometimes individuals seek hormone replacement therapy to accomplish this. Yet, while hormone therapy (such as for menopausal symptoms or for those with low testosterone) can help correct a deficiency, when you stop adding the hormones the deficiency remains. Hormone therapy doesn't cure the imbalance. I would rather restore a natural balance to the body by supporting the metabolic pathways for hormone production and metabolism. Then, if supplements are still needed, the body is in the best possible condition to use them.

Your body is talking to you, so let's honor that conversation. The best way to do that is with food. On this prescription, we will use food to:

1. Remove the barriers to hormone metabolism by stimulating enzymes to wash the receptor sites and rid the body of excess stored fat that is inhibiting proper hormone balance.

2. Repair the mechanisms for proper hormone production by feeding the glands that produce hormones with the nutrients they need. We will activate enzymes for the synthesis, conversion, and detoxification of excess hormones.

3. Restore normal hormone production and assimilation with three key lifestyle strategies.

GUIDELINES FOR YOUR HORMONE REPAIR RX

To properly follow your hormone nutrition prescription, be sure to do the following:

- You will be taking this prescription five times every day (by eating five times every day). You will have three strategic hormone-balancing meals and two targeted hormone-balancing snacks every day.

- You will take your prescription (eat) every three to four hours.

- You will split each week into two parts, eating according to one meal plan for four consecutive days and then the other plan for three consecutive days. Then you repeat the pattern.

- Typically, my clients need to stay on this prescription for a minimum of three to six months. You will notice a ton of benefits within the first thirty days, but you really need to give the body enough time to heal and create a new homeostasis.

- If you object to any of the foods for any reason, just replace them with a different food from the Foundational Foods List or the Top 20 Power Foods for Hormone Repair list. For example, you could substitute oranges for pineapples or eggs for wild salmon.

- Read this entire prescription before starting, and be sure to review the Self-Discovery Zone periodically to assess your progress. Keep in mind there might be other pathways in other chapters that need nurturing, too, and that could be related to your hormone imbalance.

- It's not uncommon for my clients to express their hormonal concerns to their doctors and to be offered a prescription for hormone replacement therapy as the primary or sole option for relief. This is quite often done without ever calling for any lab testing, and doctors tend to say things like, "Hormones fluctuate so labs are useless." I'm a real stickler on this one. It is *always* important to get stable baseline values before introducing any hormones into the system in any form. That includes birth control pills, pellets, patches, and IUDs, as well as progestin or testosterone creams, injectables, and Viagra. Once you start disrupting the hormones from the outside, it becomes difficult to know what is normal for you. For this reason, I urge you to engage your doctor about starting this program, and request those labs anyway. Put it in writing, with the reason you want the lab (i.e., your symptoms) next to the request. It's easy—just go back to the Self-Discovery Zone. Once you have that baseline, tell your doctor you would like to use food therapy to maximize your body's ability to stabilize your hormones before trying replacement therapy. You only want to replace what you really need. Don't forget to drink half your body weight in ounces of spring water every day, with a maximum of 100 ounces per day.

EAT YOUR MEDICINE: YOUR HORMONE REPAIR RX

To begin, here is your Top 20 Power Foods list. Use these foods in addition to the foods on the Foundational Foods List to power-up your hormone repair food prescription.

This prescription has two parts, with two distinctively different meal maps. Follow the first map for four consecutive days, then switch to the second meal map for the last three days of the week. Do this for as long as you are following this prescription. Do not alter the order and categories as they are laid out—there is method to my madness!

My strategy during the first four days is to add therapeutic levels of healthy fats as building blocks for hormone production, while layering in high-fiber,

Apples

Avocados

Beets

Black pepper

Blueberries

Broccoli

Cabbage

Cinnamon

Eggs, whole (not just whites), organic

Flaxseed

Garlic

Ginger, fresh or ground

Legumes

Olive oil

Oranges

Pineapples

Nuts, raw

Sweet potatoes

Turmeric

Salmon, wild-caught

cellulose-rich veggies that stimulate enzymes to wash the receptor sites and convert food into micronutrients for hormone metabolism.

MEAL MAP FOR HORMONE REPAIR, DAYS 1–4

BREAKFAST	SNACK	LUNCH	SNACK	DINNER
Protein	Protein	Protein	Protein	Protein
Vegetable	Vegetable	Vegetable	Vegetable	Vegetable
Healthy Fat	Healthy Fat	Healthy Fat		

During the last three days of the week, my strategy is to add natural sugars from fruits and complex carbs to support the adaptation hormones of the adrenals and the insulin, leptin, and adiponectin feedback loop with the fat cells, stimulating the fat metabolism to manufacture hormones and creating a homeostasis in the metabolic pathways for hormone repair.

MEAL MAP FOR HORMONE REPAIR, DAYS 5–7

BREAKFAST	SNACK	LUNCH	SNACK	DINNER
Protein Vegetable Fruit (low G.I.) Complex Carb	Protein Vegetable	Protein Vegetable Fruit (low G.I.)	Protein Vegetable	Protein Vegetable Complex Carb

A DAY IN THE LIFE OF HORMONE REPAIR

Now let's take a closer look at how you might implement this prescription. You can mix and match however you like, and you can keep your meals as basic as you want or get as elaborate as you want, as long as you follow the meal maps. Focus on the power foods and layer in additional items from the Foundational Foods List. As long as you stay true to the meal maps, you're going to experience success.

To get you started, here is a sample day for the first four days of the week, with corresponding recipes for breakfast, lunch, and dinner, and some great snack ideas (recipes provided appear in boldface in the meal maps). This is an actual day created for one of my clients.

SAMPLE DAY FOR HORMONE REPAIR, DAYS 1–4

BREAKFAST	SNACK	LUNCH	SNACK	DINNER
Green Smoothie	Nitrate-free deli turkey slices with green pepper strips and ¼ cup raw almonds	**Shrimp Salad**	Chicken slices wrapped in romaine lettuce	**Grilled New York Strip Steak**

RECIPES

These recipes use the power foods periodically in addition to the core Foundational Foods List. As you spend more time on this prescription, you will discover your own great recipes (or explore the ones on my website). Incorporate the power foods into your plan as often as you can, but also remember that adherence to the style and food categories is an equally important part of this prescription.

GREEN SMOOTHIE
Serves 2

  1 English cucumber, chopped
  1 Granny Smith apple, cored and chopped
  4 cups fresh baby spinach
  1 cup almond milk
  1 cup cold water
  2 tablespoons chia seeds
  $1/2$ teaspoon stevia, plus more to taste
  Juice of $1/2$ lemon

In a blender, combine all the ingredients and blend until smooth. If you don't have a powerful blender, pulse the ingredients two at a time, then combine. It's best to drink the smoothie as soon as you make it, but it will also hold in the refrigerator. Consume within 8 to 12 hours.

SHRIMP SALAD
Serves 2

  1 red bell pepper
  2 teaspoons cider vinegar
  2 tablespoons olive oil
  12 ounces peeled and deveined shrimp (21–25 shrimp)
  1 tablespoon minced garlic
  1 head of butter lettuce, chopped
  $1/2$ medium avocado, sliced
  1 cup alfalfa sprouts
  $1/4$ cup thinly sliced radishes
  2 tablespoons fresh thyme
  Sea salt
  Black pepper
  $1/2$ lemon, cut into wedges

Preheat the oven to 500°F. Place the red pepper on a baking sheet and roast until the skin of the bell pepper is black and charred. Remove from the oven and use tongs to put the pepper into a paper bag, then close the bag. When cool enough to handle, remove the skin and seeds.

In a food processor, or using a knife and chopping finely, puree the roasted pepper and the vinegar.

In a large sauté pan over high heat, combine the olive oil, shrimp, and garlic. Cook for 2 to 3 minutes, or until the shrimp turn color.

In a large salad bowl, toss the lettuce, avocado, sprouts, and radishes with the shrimp and pepper puree. Sprinkle in the thyme and salt and pepper to taste. Serve with the lemon wedges.

GRILLED NEW YORK STRIP STEAK
Serves 1

$1/4$ teaspoon chili powder

$1/8$ teaspoon paprika

$1/8$ teaspoon ground coriander

$1/8$ teaspoon ground cumin

$1/8$ teaspoon dry mustard

1 teaspoon chopped fresh or $1/4$ teaspoon dried oregano

1 4-ounce strip steak

1 to 2 cups trimmed broccoli florets

Juice and grated zest of 1 lemon

Sea salt

Freshly ground black pepper

1 tablespoon chopped fresh parsley

Preheat a grill or heat a cast-iron skillet over high heat.

Combine the chili powder, paprika, coriander, cumin, and mustard in a small mixing bowl. Coat the steak with the spices. Grill or sauté the steak until the internal temperature reaches 130°F for rare, 135°F for medium, 145°F for medium well, and 155°F for well done. Remove the steak from the grill and let rest.

Cook the broccoli on the grill for 2 to 3 minutes, or just until tender. Place in a bowl and squeeze half the lemon juice on the broccoli, then season with $1/2$ teaspoon salt and pepper to taste. Toss with the lemon zest and sprinkle with remaining lemon juice.

Garnish the steak with the parsley and serve with the lemon and broccoli.

MORNING SNACK

On these days, remember to choose a healthy fat, vegetable, and protein for your snack.

- Romaine lettuce wrap containing avocado slices and cooked chicken
- Celery sticks—fill two with almond butter and two with hummus
- Small spinach salad topped with strips of leftover steak and drizzled with olive oil and balsamic vinegar

AFTERNOON SNACK

As the meal map states, this snack should contain only a protein and a vegetable.

- Nitrate-free deli turkey wrapped around bell pepper strips
- Leftover steak cut into strips and dipped in salsa
- Small bowl of lentil soup, topped with shredded carrots and celery

SAMPLE DAY FOR HORMONE REPAIR, DAYS 5–7

BREAKFAST	SNACK	LUNCH	SNACK	DINNER
Poached Egg Sandwich with Blueberries	Turkey jerky and baby carrots	**Grilled Chicken and Vegetable Stew with Melon**	Hard-boiled eggs and green pepper strips	**Steak Fried Rice**

RECIPES

POACHED EGG SANDWICH WITH BLUEBERRIES

Serves 1

2 teaspoons white vinegar

2 large eggs

2 cups baby spinach

Sea salt

Freshly ground black pepper

$1/2$ sprouted-grain or spelt bagel

Dash of Tabasco (optional)

1 teaspoon nutritional yeast (optional)

1 cup fresh blueberries

Heat enough water in a deep 2-quart saucepan to come 1 inch up the side. Add the vinegar and bring to a simmer over medium heat. One at a time, crack the eggs into a custard cup or small ramekin, then use the handle of a spatula or spoon to quickly stir the water in one direction until it's spinning. Carefully drop the egg into the center of the water; the swirling water will help prevent the white from "feathering," or spreading out in the pan. After adding both eggs, turn off the heat, cover the pan, and set a timer for 5 minutes. Leave undisturbed to poach.

Heat a medium sauté pan over high heat, then add the spinach and $1/4$ cup water. Season to taste with salt and pepper, and cook the spinach 2 to 3 minutes, until wilted.

Toast the bagel half, if desired.

Place the spinach and poached eggs on the bagel. Sprinkle with Tabasco and nutritional yeast. Serve with blueberries on the side.

GRILLED CHICKEN AND VEGETABLE STEW

Serves 4

3 cups chicken broth

$1/4$ head green cabbage, cored and sliced

1 carrot, diced

$1/2$ cup sliced yellow onion

1 celery rib, diced

1 tablespoon minced garlic

$1/8$ teaspoon celery seed, ground in a spice grinder

3 cups chopped ripe tomatoes

Pinch of cayenne pepper

Sea salt

Freshly ground black pepper

4 bone-in, skin-on chicken thighs (1 pound total)

1 tablespoon chili powder

1 tablespoon chopped fresh parsley

Place the chicken broth in a stockpot set over high heat and bring to a boil. Reduce to a simmer and add the cabbage, carrot, onion, celery, garlic, ground celery seed, tomatoes, cayenne, 1/2 teaspoon salt, and 1/4 teaspoon pepper. Cook for 20 minutes.

Meanwhile, preheat a gas or charcoal grill until very hot.

Place the chicken in a bowl or plastic bag, add the chili powder, and stir to coat the chicken with the seasoning. Season the chicken with a little salt and pepper, then grill skin side down for 6 to 8 minutes. Turn and grill on the other side for another 5 minutes, or until the internal temperature reaches 165°F.

Spoon the vegetables onto a plate and top each serving with 1 chicken thigh. Sprinkle with parsley and serve.

STEAK FRIED RICE

Serves 4

3/4 cup uncooked barley
1/2 cup uncooked wild rice
1 1-pound boneless sirloin steak, cut into 1/2-inch cubes
Sea salt
Freshly ground black pepper
1/2 cup beef broth
3/4 cup thinly sliced celery
1 cup thinly sliced carrots
1/2 cup fresh or frozen snow peas
1 tablespoon minced garlic
2 teaspoons grated fresh ginger
2 teaspoons rice wine vinegar
1/4 teaspoon red pepper flakes
3 tablespoons tamari
1/4 cup thinly sliced green onions

Place the barley and 3 cups of water in a saucepan over high heat and bring to a boil. Reduce the heat to a simmer, cover, and cook the barley until tender and most of the liquid has been absorbed, 20 to 25 minutes. Let stand 5 minutes.

Place 2 cups of water in another saucepan over high heat and bring to a boil. Add the wild rice and reduce the heat to a simmer. Cover and cook until tender, 20 to 25 minutes. Drain.

Season the steak with salt and pepper. In a large sauté pan set over high heat, cook the steak until nicely browned on all sides, 2 to 3 minutes. Remove the steak.

Add the beef broth to the sauté pan and bring to a boil, stirring to loosen any browned bits on the bottom of the pan. Add the celery, carrots, snow peas, garlic, and ginger, and cook until all the liquid is absorbed. Add the barley and wild rice, and cook for 1 minute to heat through. Add the vinegar, red pepper flakes, tamari, and steak. Season to taste, stirring, and cook for 2 to 3 minutes more. Serve, garnished with the green onions.

SNACK IDEAS FOR HORMONE REPAIR, DAYS 5–7

Both morning and afternoon snacks should contain a protein and a vegetable:

- Nitrate-free deli turkey and broccoli florets
- Hard-boiled eggs chopped with celery and pickles
- Steak strips wrapped in romaine lettuce leaves
- Mashed cooked white beans, spread on cucumber slices
- Fresh kale salad with chickpeas

RESTORE HORMONAL BALANCE: TOP THREE NON-FOOD STRATEGIES

Your food prescription is always top priority, but there are many tweaks you can make to improve your hormone manufacture and metabolism. Add some or all of these to your daily routine on top of your food prescription, and you will boost your body's ability to regulate and balance your hormones.

LIGHT CARDIO + HEAVY WEIGHTS

When you are balancing your hormones, the key is light cardio but heavy weights twice a week, in short bursts, to stabilize and support the adrenals. By doing this, you are invoking the hormones of repair in the body by creating microtrauma in the muscles. This lowers the crisis hormones and stimulates the rebuild, repair, and restoration hormones. You want to keep the cardio in as well, so as to promote blood flow and the lymphatic flushing of the muscle, so your tissue doesn't get too acidic. Also, developing muscle by lifting weights causes the fat cells to break down, and that is helpful with this prescription because less excess fat means less excess hormone production.

ACTIVE STRESS REDUCTION

While some prescriptions require more passive stress-reduction techniques, hormone repair calls for active stress reduction. Journaling, mind mapping, yoga, meditation, biofeedback, EMDR (Eye Movement Desensitization and Reprocessing), neurofeedback, and talk therapy are all excellent ways to manage stress in the face of hormonal imbalance. Pick your favorites and try to do something stress-relieving every day—anything whereby you take an active role in relieving your own stress. Make this an appointment on your calendar—it is that important. Active stress reduction engages the cognitive brain and helps to repattern the thought processes, which can be an anchor for sex, stress, and brain hormone rebalancing.

PRACTICING JOY

Experiencing joy can make a profound difference to your hormone balance. Surprised? Every time you stimulate the feel-good hormones, they help open and revitalize your hormone metabolism pathways. So for this prescription, I recommend watching comedies, telling jokes, having tickle sessions, singing, and doing anything else you really love to do. For me, horseback riding brings joy. So, find that thing you love to do; if you think you don't have time for it, make it a *priority* in your life. It can be as simple as meeting a friend for lunch who always makes you laugh, or Googling funny memes online, or as complex as taking up an intricate hobby that makes the time fly by and puts you in a good mood.

BRIEFING YOUR DREAM TEAM

Some doctors may say that hormone tests aren't necessary because the results change so often. It's true that hormones fluctuate. There is a range of normal values for the sex hormones in women, depending on where they are in the monthly cycle, or even whether or not they are still having a cycle. If you always test at the same point in your cycle, you can get a good idea of any deficiencies, excesses, and trends. My ideal when checking sex hormones, for those still cycling, is to check three days after the onset of the period.

These are the tests I recommend. Remember to write down your official request along with your symptoms:

- **E2, or estradiol tests:** An estradiol test measures the amount of estrogen in your blood. Estradiol helps with the growth of the female sex organs and controls the way fat is distributed in the female body. In men, it helps with fertility and sex drive. This test checks how well the ovaries or adrenal glands are functioning.

- **Testosterone tests, both free and total:** This blood test measures the level of testosterone your body is producing. It can help diagnose conditions like decreased sex drive and infertility in both genders.

- **Sex hormone–binding globulin, or SHBG test:** This is a carrier protein that indicates how hormones are being transported in the body and being delivered to receptor sites. Low levels of SHBG can relate to obesity and type 2 diabetes, while high levels can relate to hyperthyroidism and/or low testosterone.

- **Vitamin D test:** This test reports the levels of vitamin D in the blood. It can help diagnose or monitor issues that occur with vitamin D deficiency, like bone weakness and poor food absorption.

- **FSH test:** This test measures your level of follicle-stimulating hormone, which is what helps manage a woman's menstrual cycle and stimulates the ovaries to produce eggs. Testing for FSH can help diagnose menopause or problems in becoming pregnant. FSH also stimulates the production of sperm in men, and can point to problems with male infertility.

- **LH test:** This measures the luteinizing hormone (LH), and is useful even in postmenopausal women. LH is produced by the pituitary gland in the brain. It aids in the release of eggs during the menstrual cycle and can help pinpoint when you are ovulating. Some people believe you

For most of the lab tests mentioned in this book, the ranges considered normal or abnormal by the lab analyzing the sample will tell you whether you need to be concerned about those values or discuss them with your doctor. There is one exception, however, and that is vitamin D. There are varying opinions on what constitutes a normal vitamin D level. Typically, individuals with healthy hormone metabolism have levels between 50 and 80 ng/mL, but many labs don't consider hormone homeostasis in their evaluation and accept as normal levels that are under 50. You could be told your vitamin D level of 30 is "normal." However, I believe that for ideal hormone metabolism and hormone repair, vitamin D levels should range between 50 and 80.

can't have an LH surge if you're not ovulating, but this number can indicate pituitary homeostasis, even in postmenopausal women, so insist on it.

- **Progesterone test:** This hormone is produced mainly in the ovaries and works in concert with estrogen to balance the hormonal cycle. Progesterone levels rise and fall on a monthly basis.

- **C-reactive protein (CRP) and homocysteine tests:** These two tests are typically used to determine cardiovascular risk, but they also are signs of inflammation and hormonal imbalance, especially in men.

SOMETHING TO CHEW ON

Hormones are rhythmic. Women obviously have a monthly cycle before they reach menopause, but even women who are postmenopausal and don't ovulate anymore still have hormonal cycles. Many postmenopausal women still report a change in vaginal discharge, breast tenderness, sleep patterns, and libido throughout the month—many of the same changes that happen when an individual is cycling. Men have hormonal cycles that seem to be much more seasonal, but the cycles exist.

Tracking this rhythm can tell a lot. I am a strong proponent of using apps or a calendar to chart your cycle and symptoms. Hormone imbalances typically have trends, and if you can start to see those trends in your body, you can know where to back off a little bit and when to go for a full-court press. For example, I am extra diligent in the second half of my cycle because, post-ovulation, that seems to be when my body ebbs more significantly and I experience more hormonal symptoms—so that's when I really step up the power foods. Being aware of these cycles and charting the trends of these cycles will allow you to preemptively support your body so that the cycles become opportunities to flourish, not to flounder.

CHAPTER 8

High Cholesterol, Inflammation, and Other Signs of Impaired Lipid Metabolism

Maybe you are under the impression that fat and cholesterol are bad things. Actually, fat is good and cholesterol is biochemical gold. Without cholesterol circulating in our bloodstream, we would lose our minds, and then we would die. The body's entire system would fail and shut down. So thank goodness for cholesterol! We need some level of cholesterol circulating in our bloodstream all the time.

But what we don't need is too much of it, especially in the presence of inflammation. The exact value that represents a healthy level of serum cholesterol will probably be debated for centuries, but what science is now saying is that cholesterol becomes more harmful in the presence of inflammation, because inflammation is what makes it stick to the arterial walls. Inflammation acts like the glove to receive the pitch; when cholesterol starts sticking to the arteries and hardening, this becomes a risk factor for heart disease. The immune system regulates inflammation and the adrenals regulate inflammation, so this is one reason a lot of individuals with inflammation that is causing other problems (like autoimmunity or depression, for example) seem to be at an increased risk for heart disease as well.

But saying we should not *eat* fat and cholesterol if we have high serum cholesterol or because we want to prevent high cholesterol is like saying we should get rid of all the water in the world just because we had a flood—or in case we might get a flood sometime in the future. Of course, we can't get rid of all the water; we need water or we will die. When water levels on earth are high, you find ways to capture and utilize that valuable resource, to get it back to the places it needs to go, rather than letting it overrun the land. This is why we build dams and reservoirs or install water tanks and water towers. This is why we build bridges and tunnels to go over or under waterways, and we use water treatment plants to make use of the water we've captured. Yes, a flood can be destructive, and cholesterol can be destructive, but water and cholesterol are both life-giving, valuable resources.

An elevated cholesterol reading is not a sign that you are eating too much cholesterol or fats. It is a sign that you are having a problem metabolizing cholesterol. You aren't using this extremely valuable substance to fuel your hormone production.

What we're talking about is lipid metabolism, and there are other considerations as well. Triglycerides, which are made of one fat molecule and three sugar molecules, are an indication that the body is struggling to metabolize sugar. An elevated triglyceride level, then, is a huge warning sign that the body is heading toward a diabetic state. And this is something that doesn't respond well to pharmaceutical intervention. When the body begins to bind sugars with fat, rather than utilizing those sugars, this can cause the blood to become sticky. However, stabilizing the blood sugar throughout the day by eating in a particular style (as with this prescription) seems to bring down elevated triglycerides better than any other method.

When you are not metabolizing lipids as you should, your body will talk to you by generating some pretty uncomfortable symptoms, such as hormone imbalance, memory and cognition issues, depression, and diabetes, as well as coronary heart disease. In fact, people with problems related to cholesterol metabolism probably account for 50 percent of my practice. We need cholesterol to function and thrive, and all of what the body manufactures from cholesterol is almost unbelievable. All of the sex hormones, brain chemistry, hormones that regulate blood sugar and blood pressure, the immune hormones, the hormones that manage inflammation, and hormones that allow the body to adapt to stress—these are just a few examples of what cholesterol makes possible in the body.

A lot of people will say that if you have high cholesterol, all you need to do is take a medication and move on with your life. However, pooling cholesterol in the bloodstream is such a significant fork in the road for your health that repairing it should be a *top priority*, and medicating it should *only be done in a crisis situation*. Elevated serum cholesterol is the one serious health situation for which medication is prescribed almost nonchalantly. And yet, cholesterol metabolism—or lack of it—can manifest in a significant number of chronic diseases. This is not something to brush off or play around with. This is serious business.

High blood levels of cholesterol mean there's a cholesterol metabolism deficiency. If you don't metabolize cholesterol well, or if you don't produce enough of it, or if you inhibit cholesterol production by a medication, you can develop high blood pressure, low serum vitamin D, poor bile acid production, and poor dietary fat metabolism, the latter which causes increased fat storage. The human body typically responds to this kind of situation by creating more pro-inflammatory hormones. This leads to plaque in the arteries and even what they are calling "sludge" in the brain, causing things like dementia, Alzheimer's disease, and memory and cognition issues. These conditions can all eventually lead to heart disease and stroke.

But here's the part I love: Cholesterol metabolism is entirely *nutrient dependent!* Yep, we've got this one. Doctors and scientists know this very well, but the nutrition prescription that's often given is to eliminate fat and cholesterol from the diet. And let me tell you—that is the wrong, wrong, wrong prescription for your health.

Lowering serum cholesterol by reducing cholesterol consumption to prevent coronary heart disease (as many popular books and doctors advise) leaves out the part about your being a dynamic body. You need memory, cognition, immunity, and all the other abilities listed earlier that cholesterol does for you. I always love to see doctors focusing more on food than on medication, but you can't focus on the E and ignore the M. Removing cholesterol and fat from the diet doesn't repair the why—why the body isn't metabolizing cholesterol. And, it also shortchanges you from realizing all the incredible health benefits you get when you convert that biochemical gold.

We must use food to repair the metabolic pathways for cholesterol metabolism so you can unearth that gem called cholesterol.

THE SELF-DISCOVERY ZONE

There are many different signs that you could be dealing with issues of metabolizing cholesterol. The signs are wide-ranging because cholesterol metabolism influences so many different hormone pathways, but here are a few of the clearest signs:

- Appetite that is out of control

- Blood pressure that is too high

- Bone density that is too low, or a diagnosis of osteoporosis or osteopenia

- Diabetes or prediabetes diagnosis (also see Chapter 10)

- Earlobe creases

- Fat accumulation around your belly, abdomen, and/or waist (like a pot belly, spare tire, or muffin top)—not being able to zip up your jeans

- HDL serum cholesterol levels that are too low

- Hormonal issues, including low sex drive, menstrual irregularities, impotence, infertility, and PCOS (also see Chapter 10)

- LDL serum cholesterol levels that are too high

- Serum vitamin D levels that are too low

- Skin that becomes dry, especially around the lips and on the elbows

- Sweat resistance—you don't sweat easily during exercise

- Testosterone levels that are too low

- Triglycerides that are too high

- Water retention—your socks, watch, and rings are leaving marks

DEALING, NOT HEALING

Cholesterol is a big issue in our society. Many years ago, scary studies came out that linked an elevated serum cholesterol level to coronary heart disease. In fact, the top risk factors for coronary heart disease are (notice they are all, with the possible exception of smoking, related to imbalances in metabolic pathways):

- Smoking

- High blood cholesterol

- High blood pressure

- Physical inactivity

- Obesity or being overweight

- Diabetes

Many times, the first line of defense for high cholesterol was to treat it with statin drugs, to mute it in the bloodstream. But the fact that we are simply muting it is scary indeed. Cholesterol-lowering medication doesn't solve the cholesterol metabolism problem. If it did, people could take it for a period of time, and then stop, and they would be healed. It just makes the lab tests look better; it's a transient fix. That's why we aren't realizing the benefits of the drugs we thought we would see. Despite better lab values, cholesterol medication is not the savior we had all hoped it would be; it is no longer strongly associated with a reduced risk of heart disease, which kind of defeats the whole purpose of the drug.

With my clients, the medication was especially concerning, given its strong side effects. The National Institutes of Health has stated that the side effects can include intestinal problems, liver damage, muscle inflammation, memory loss, mental confusion, and elevated blood sugar, and its use can also stimulate the onset of type 2 diabetes.

Fortunately, when it comes to high cholesterol, elevated triglycerides, and heart disease, I have found in my clinical experience that doctors are much more receptive to nutritional strategies. I don't always agree with their nutritional advice, but at least the door is open for a dialogue. Sometimes I say to a doctor, "Just give me forty-five days," or "Just give me ninety days without medical intervention. Let me try to reverse this situation nutritionally."

That's because I am always highly motivated to keep my clients off statin drugs. Statin drugs have one main function: *They specifically block the production of cholesterol in the liver.* Now, you might think that sounds good, but what if I were to replace the word *cholesterol* in that statement with the definition of what cholesterol does in the body—the building block for all steroid hormones. The new sentence would read: *Statins specifically block the production of your sex hormones, your memory and cognition, and your ability to regulate your blood sugar and immunity.*

Yikes! Would you touch that drug with a ten-foot pole? Cholesterol is the building block for all those things, so if that's what statins really do, we don't want anything to do with them. We have to find a better way.

WHAT SCIENCE SAYS IS TRUE

There is a longstanding misconception that eating cholesterol causes high serum cholesterol, but the research doesn't support this. There is a raging debate about whether high serum cholesterol equates to an increased rate of cardiovascular disease; my opinion on this is that it depends. It seems that a combination of elevated serum cholesterol, inflammation, and lack of certain enzymes creates that perfect cardiovascular storm. But if and when we repair cholesterol metabolism, we won't need to worry whether or not elevated cholesterol causes heart disease—because we will be converting cholesterol into health.

A recent review of research states that epidemiological data have clearly demonstrated *that dietary cholesterol is not correlated with increased risk for coronary heart disease,*[*] and while some individuals are particularly sensitive to cholesterol (about 25 percent of the population) and do experience a rise in "bad" LDL cholesterol with increased intake of dietary cholesterol, they also experience a simultaneous rise in "good" HDL cholesterol. The review concludes with a recommendation that limiting dietary cholesterol should be reconsidered.

_____

* M. L. Fernandez, "Rethinking Dietary Cholesterol," *Current Opinion in Clinical Nutritional and Metabolic Care* 15, no. 2 (March 2012): 117–21.

TARGETED PATHWAYS FOR REPAIR

Cholesterol metabolism happens in the liver. When the liver becomes stressed by too much toxic material it has to filter out, it can stop paying attention to cholesterol metabolism. At that point, cholesterol can back up and start pooling in the bloodstream. In some people with a genetic inability to detoxify efficiently, the problem becomes even worse (I am one of these people). For example, those who have glutathione deficiency (a deficiency in certain enzymes, associated with liver detoxification) or 5MTHFR (a genetic inability to fully metabolize folate) have a tendency toward elevated cholesterol production when the liver is struggling. Individuals with bowel problems or GI problems like leaky gut (whereby food particles leak out of injuries in the mucosal lining) can have enhanced absorption of cholesterol in the intestines, so consumed cholesterol might be absorbed too rapidly, leading to high blood cholesterol levels. Individuals who suffer from food allergies have a tendency to have increased cholesterol absorption through intestines as well, and may also have cholesterol levels in the blood that are too high.

The problem with cholesterol in the bloodstream is that once it's there, the body has to break it down. If it's being delivered too quickly and the liver can't keep up, or if the liver is blocked by doing other jobs, the problem gets worse and worse, and the serum cholesterol levels go up and up.

And that's bad. When we stop metabolizing cholesterol, a few things start to happen:

- Bad cholesterol begins to pool instead of being metabolized into the hormones that stimulate mood, energy, sex hormone production, blood sugar stabilization, immune function, blood pressure regulation, and body structure development and repair.

- Good cholesterol begins to decline, creating the demand for hormone-like pro-inflammatory substances (prostaglandins) and inhibiting sex hormone uptake.

- Immune modulation, or the immune system's ability to adapt, becomes compromised, which increases fat cell accumulation, reducing memory and cognition.

- Production of bile salts is compromised, lowering the body's ability to break down fats and cholesterol molecules, which then creates a deficiency in hormones and vitamin D, and adversely affects brain chemistry, signaling the body to slow cholesterol metabolism even further.

We often see this dysfunction start to develop when women go through menopause. They begin to have hormone imbalances and changes in their lipid profiles, whether it's a higher LDL (bad) cholesterol level, or a lower HDL (good) cholesterol level, or an elevated total cholesterol, or an elevated CRP (indicating inflammation)—or all of these. They are red flags. But the message is not to tweak the hormones or the inflammation or the blood cholesterol. That's treating the problem downstream. The message is to go to the source—to improve cholesterol metabolism so that these processes can regulate themselves. And if you and your doctor decide that medication is necessary in your particular case, this can give that medication the best possible chance of working.

REMOVE, REPAIR, AND RESTORE

Our goal together is to support healthy production of cholesterol, adequate absorption, efficient removal of excess, and a balancing of the metabolic pathways that convert cholesterol into the steroid hormones. We will nourish and support the liver in particular by providing the micronutrients it needs and by freeing up the body's other detoxification systems, so the liver can do its job. Specifically, we will:

1. Remove obstacles in the liver and in the body's detoxification pathways to promote healthy cholesterol metabolism, so you can make all the hormones you need to thrive. We're going to take that cholesterol and spin straw into gold!

2. Repair the metabolic pathways for lipid metabolism in the body and also repair inflammation that can happen in the mucosal lining when cholesterol pools in the blood.

3. Restore the body's natural ability to produce cholesterol appropriately through easy lifestyle interventions.

GUIDELINES FOR YOUR LIPID METABOLISM REPAIR RX

To properly follow your cholesterol metabolism prescription, be sure to do the following:

- You will be taking this prescription six times every day (by eating six times every day). That's three meals and three snacks. You will also be eating one meal plan for the entire seven days of each week.

- If you have a recent diagnosis of high cholesterol and your doctor thinks you should go on medication, try to get your doctor to allow you ninety days on a nutrition program, checking labs at the halfway mark, to see if the imbalance is corrected without pharmaceuticals. In particularly concerning cases, your doctor might want to check your lipid panel every four weeks until it stabilizes. This may also be the case if your doctor is attempting to guide you through medication removal (as in cases in which the patient is starting to exhibit memory and cognition effects, which sometimes happens with statin drugs).

- Typically, my clients need to stay on this prescription for three to six months. After that, I have them cycle in one month of this prescription four times a year, to keep and maintain those open pathways. Your body won't be able to fully restore metabolic pathways for cholesterol metabolism more quickly than this, so keep it up for the duration and you will get your cholesterol levels safe and stable.

- If you object to any of the foods for any reason, just replace them with a different food from the Foundational Foods List or the Top 20 Power Foods for Cholesterol Metabolism Repair list. For example, you could substitute carrots for spinach or pork for sardines or other seafood.

- Tell your doctor before you start this program. To get the most out of your time and to prove your progress, ask for the lab tests I recommend at the end of this chapter, then repeat them after you do this prescription to see if your doctor still thinks you need medication. Ask your doctor to give you ninety days to get your cholesterol down before trying statins. Some doctors want to recheck in forty-five days and I'm game. Say you are specifically trying to tackle this, and your doctor will likely be all for it.

- Drink half your body weight in ounces of spring water every day, with a maximum of 100 ounces.

EAT YOUR MEDICINE: YOUR LIPID METABOLISM RX

Let's begin with your list of power foods for tackling high cholesterol, inflammation, and impaired lipid metabolism. Use these foods as much as you can in addition to selecting from the Foundational Foods List for this prescription. When you particularly emphasize these foods and incorporate them into your meals and snacks whenever you can, you will help feed the pathways for cholesterol metabolism.

TOP 20 POWER FOODS FOR CHOLESTEROL METABOLISM REPAIR

Avocados

Green beans

Berries, such as raspberries, blueberries, blackberries

Carrots

Fish—any kind

Garlic

Legumes—lentils, black beans, kidney beans, chickpeas

Mushrooms

Oats

Onions

Oranges

Pears

Pork—lean and nitrite free

Prunes

Radishes

Rosemary

Sardines

Spinach

Tomatoes

Walnuts

Follow this meal map exactly for best results, but choose the foods you love, making liberal use of the Top 20 Power Foods list.

My strategy with this particular eating program is to stimulate the digestive enzymes that help to break down the cholesterol molecule by increasing the raw vegetable and fruit contents. Raw vegetables help to stimulate the digestive enzymes you need, and the steady supply of fruit helps to keep blood sugar stable. Both also add fiber to help pull cholesterol out of the blood and the body through the colon.

We will also stabilize your blood sugar with a steady supply of healthy fats like olive oil, avocados, and walnuts. Healthy fats in combination with raw plant food enzymes and high fiber levels elevate the amount of bile salts that support fat metabolism and regulate salt and water balance in the blood. We will also focus on taurine-rich and glycine-rich protein sources, which also help with bile production, support healthy cholesterol metabolism, and even give your brain, memory, and cognition a boost.

You will stay on this meal plan for the entire week, and repeat for as long as necessary to get your cholesterol back into balance.

MEAL MAP FOR LIPID METABOLISM REPAIR

BREAKFAST	SNACK	LUNCH	SNACK	DINNER	SNACK
Protein Complex Carb Healthy Fat Fruit (raw, high or low G.I.)	Fruit (raw, high or low G.I.) Healthy Fat	Protein Vegetable (raw, a minimum of 2 to 4 cups) Fruit (raw, high or low G.I.) Healthy Fat	Vegetable Healthy Fat	Protein Vegetable (cooked or raw, miniumum 2–4 cups) Healthy Fat	Vegetable (raw)

A DAY IN THE LIFE OF LIPID METABOLISM REPAIR

Here is an example of how you might use the Foundational Foods List to create your own meal plan using the meal map for this repair. Unlike many of the other prescriptions, you will not switch your eating style during the week; you will eat in the same balanced pattern every day. For this particular prescription, the day's rhythm and the combination of the food categories are very important.

This sample day shows how you might choose to eat during each week of your prescription, followed by recipes (as noted in boldface in the meal map) for the meals listed on this sample map.

SAMPLE DAY FOR LIPID METABOLISM REPAIRS, DAYS 1–7

BREAKFAST	SNACK	LUNCH	SNACK	DINNER	SNACK
Coconut Oats and Eggs	Orange slices sprinkled with coconut	**Steak and Spinach Salad**	Snow peas and cashews	**Pulled Pork in Collard Wrap**	Carrots

RECIPES

These recipes draw from the Top 20 Power Foods list to augment the Foundational Foods List. As you stay on this prescription, you will soon learn to create your own meals and find recipes that work in the food plan (such as those on my website). As you do this, incorporate these power foods whenever you can, but also remember that the timing of meals and the food categories for each meal are also extremely important parts of this prescription.

COCONUT OATS AND EGGS

Serves 2

4 large eggs

2 cups old-fashioned rolled oats

2 cups coconut milk

1¼ cups water

1 teaspoon stevia (optional, for more sweetness)

⅛ teaspoon sea salt

1 cup fresh blueberries

2 tablespoons sunflower seeds

¼ teaspoon ground cinnamon

Place the eggs in a small saucepan and fill with water. Bring the water to a boil over high heat, then turn off the heat and let sit for 10 minutes.

Put the oats, coconut milk, water, stevia, and salt in a medium saucepan over high heat. Bring to a boil, then reduce the heat and simmer, uncovered, for 5 minutes, stirring occasionally. Remove the pan from the heat. If desired, cover and let stand for 2 minutes before serving. (This allows the oats to absorb any remaining liquid.)

To serve, place the oatmeal in a bowl and garnish with the blueberries, sunflower seeds, and cinnamon. Serve with the hard-boiled eggs on the side.

STEAK AND SPINACH SALAD

Serves 1

4 ounces boneless sirloin steak

Sea salt

Freshly ground black pepper

2 tablespoons olive oil

1 Bosc pear, cored and sliced

$^1/_2$ red bell pepper, cored and cut into $^1/_4$-inch slices

$^1/_4$ cup thinly sliced red onion

3 cups fresh baby spinach

1 tablespoon balsamic vinegar

1 tablespoon chopped fresh parsley or cilantro

Season the steak with salt and pepper. Bring the steak to room temperature.

In a heavy-bottomed pan or cast-iron skillet, heat 1 tablespoon of the olive oil and sear the steak on both sides. Continue to cook until the internal temperature of the meat reaches 130°F for rare, 135°F for medium, 145°F for medium well, and 155°F for well done. Remove the steak from the pan and let rest for 5 minutes.

Cut the steak across the grain into $^1/_2$-inch cubes or strips.

In a mixing bowl, toss together the pear, red pepper, onion, and spinach. Add the steak, remaining tablespoon oil, and the vinegar, and toss again. Season to taste with salt and pepper, and sprinkle with parsley or coriander.

PULLED PORK IN COLLARD WRAP

Serves 6

$1^1/_2$ tablespoons chili powder

Sea salt

$^1/_2$ teaspoon ground cumin

$^1/_4$ teaspoon ground cinnamon

1 5-pound bone-in pork shoulder or butt

2 yellow onions, thinly sliced

4 garlic cloves, minced

1 cup chicken broth

Freshly ground black pepper

6 leaves collard greens

Combine the chili powder, 2 teaspoons salt, cumin, and cinnamon in a small bowl. Pat the meat dry with paper towels, then rub the spice mixture all over the pork.

Place the onions and garlic in a slow cooker, then put the meat on top and pour in the broth. Cover and slow-cook until the pork is fork-tender, 6 to 8 hours on high or 8 to 10 hours on low. Turn off the slow cooker and move the pork to a cutting board.

Set a fine-mesh strainer over a medium heatproof bowl. Pour the braising mixture from the slow cooker through the strainer, then return the solids to the cooker. Set the strained liquid aside.

When meat is cool enough to handle, use two forks to shred the meat into bite-size pieces, discarding any large pieces of fat. Measure 6 cups of shredded meat and place the remaining cooked meat in a refrigerator or freezer container for another use. Return the 6 cups of shredded meat to the slow cooker. Slowly add as much of the reserved liquid to the slow cooker as will moisten the meat. Season to taste with additional salt and pepper.

Prepare an ice bath by adding ice cubes and water to a mixing bowl. Bring a large pot filled with water to a boil over high heat. Add the collard greens and cook for 1 minute, then remove and immediately place in the ice bath. Once the leaves have cooled, remove them from the ice bath and pat dry.

Place a spoonful of meat in the center of each collard leaf, then tuck in the ends and roll up. Serve immediately.

MORNING SNACK

Note that all morning snacks should include a raw fruit and a healthy fat, according to your meal map.

- Blueberries and almonds
- Apple slices spread with almond butter
- Pineapple and shredded coconut

AFTERNOON SNACK

As you can see, all afternoon snacks should include a vegetable and a healthy fat.

- Raw carrot sticks and raw almonds
- Small spinach salad dressed with olive oil
- Celery and bell pepper with hummus

EVENING SNACK

The meal map calls for an evening snack of raw vegetables, such as the following:

- Cucumber slices
- Celery sticks
- Broccoli and cauliflower florets

RESTORE HEALTHY LIPID METABOLISM: TOP THREE NON-FOOD STRATEGIES

Food is the best way to heal cholesterol metabolism and help detoxify the body, but there are some lifestyle strategies that can add power and punch to your prescription. Try my favorites:

- **Confuse it to lose it with exercise.** Rotate your exercise style through cardio, strength training, and relaxation during the week, and don't exercise more than four days each week. If you are someone who exercises more than this, try to at least give your body some days of rest and restoration. This is so important for cholesterol repair. If you are working out like crazy and your cholesterol is high, you have to change something, because what you're doing is not working. For example, you might do cardio on Monday and Friday, strength training on Wednesday, and something relaxing, like yoga or a relaxed walk, on the weekend. On the other days, take it easy. On exercise days, of course, don't push yourself too hard or do something you can't do safely and without stress. Remember, you are a dynamic person having a biodiverse experience and your needs will be unique to you.

- **Take fiber.** Moving your bowels is extremely important for detoxifying the body, and will take some of the burden off the liver. Fiber supplements, like a spoonful of psyllium husks, ground flaxseed, or chia seed every night before bed, can help keep everything moving along smoothly.

- **Practice left brain/right brain integration or other mental stimulation.** Mental activity stimulates the demand for the master hormone pregnenolone, and this will help to stimulate the pathways for cholesterol metabolism to meet that need. Try playing any game that requires strategizing, like chess, checkers, or even soccer. You can also do any activity that requires you to coordinate both sides of the body, like dance or yoga. Passive neurofeedback (an easy type of brain wave training) or EMDR (Eye Movement Desensitization and Reprocessing, a type of psychotherapy that is excellent for stress relief) can also be good options for the less physically inclined.

BRIEFING YOUR DREAM TEAM

When your body is talking to you, telling you that your lipids aren't balanced, you can find out more. The lab tests I suggest here are all very easy add-ons for your doctor to do. But remember, you need to give your doctor reasons to run them. Go back to your Self-Discovery Zone and make a list in writing of the symptoms you are experiencing. Line them up with the lab tests you are requesting or that your doctor may already want to order during your annual physical, and get the inside scoop on your lipids. Of course, if you have high blood cholesterol, your doctor knows this because you have already had a total cholesterol test, with LDL and HDL cholesterol and triglycerides measured. There are other tests that can be illuminating, however. Ask your doctor to run these, also:

- **C-reactive protein (CRP) test:** This measures inflammation, which is now regarded as a cardiovascular risk factor and can be related to high serum cholesterol levels.

- **Aldosterone test:** This is good especially for people who have hypertension, to indicate if it is adrenal based or not. Aldosterone is a hormone released by the adrenal glands that helps the body regulate blood pressure. If your levels of this hormone are not within the normal range, it can lead to things like hard-to-control blood pressure or low blood pressure upon standing. Your levels also vary when standing, sitting, and lying down and according to your sodium intake, so ask your doctor about the results.

- **ACTH levels:** This is useful when hypertension is involved. This adrenocorticotropic hormone is released from the pituitary gland in the brain. It helps regulate blood pressure and blood sugar levels. This test can help pinpoint if your pituitary and adrenal glands are overproducing or under producing it.

- **APOE:** This is a genetic test that can indicate an inherited greater susceptibility to heart disease. Everyone has two APOE genes. Two APOE-3 genes are considered normal, but having one or two APOE-4 genes is associated with inefficient fat metabolism.

- **Fasting blood sugar, along with fasting insulin level:** These tests require you to not eat at least eight hours prior to the blood draw, and they screen for diabetes and prediabetes. These are important to look at because elevated triglycerides are a marker for the onset of prediabetes or diabetes.

- **Vitamin D:** When levels are low, it can indicate hormonal imbalances. This test can help diagnose or monitor issues that occur with vitamin D deficiency, like bone weakness and poor food absorption.

- **Hormones:** Tests of estrogen, progesterone, E2, total testosterone, and free testosterone are helpful. Cholesterol is the primary building block for these sex hormones, which are produced from metabolized cholesterol. If you aren't metabolizing cholesterol, these pathways may be disrupted, causing other problems.

- **Apolipoprotein A:** This is a protein carried in HDL, or the "good," cholesterol. It helps with the process of removing "bad" cholesterol from your body, reducing your cardiovascular risk.

SOMETHING TO CHEW ON

The biggest paradigm shift comes when addressing cholesterol or lipid issues, and the solution is to look at the big picture, the whole body, and long-term goals. It's easy to get hung up on and/or terrified by that little number, and feel pressured to start statin therapy immediately. But remember that we aren't studying for one test that we need to pass; we are studying food together to improve your whole life. Instead of focusing on that one scary number, focus on the *why*. Why are you pooling cholesterol in your bloodstream and how can you resolve this?

Some people don't take that little number seriously at all. They say, "Oh, my cholesterol is high, so I guess I should take this drug." Don't take this lightly! This is not a nonchalant therapy.

I often ask clients, "Why are you on statins?"

"Because my cholesterol is 248!"

"Let's fix that," I say.

"I thought I was fixing it," they say.

Never forget that your body is talking to you. Even doctors forget this. I had a doctor that came to see me as a client, and I said, "Any health issues?"

"Nope, not really," he said. We continued to talk. And then he said, "Oh, well, I have been taking statin drugs for the last eight years."

"So you have high cholesterol?" I said.

"No, I don't have high cholesterol," he said.

"Then stop taking the drug," I said.

"But then I will have high cholesterol," he said.

"You have a cholesterol metabolism problem," I said. "So let's fix it. You are too young and have too much life left in you to have this problem, and I want you around for a long time so you can come help my clients!"

We got his level down, he went off the drugs, and now he sends me all his patients who have high cholesterol.

So let's quit fixing the test and start fixing the metabolic pathways. Let's start fixing *you*.

CHAPTER 9

Mood Changes and Cognitive Challenges

The brain is our final frontier, of sorts. It is complex and diverse and in many ways is unfathomable. Dysfunction in the brain can manifest in different ways with different symptoms, both transitory and permanent, and it can be intimidating to try to do anything about that—from mood changes like depression or anxiety to cognitive issues like brain fog, memory problems, attention problems, or dyslexia. Even doctors say they aren't completely sure why medications prescribed for mood and cognitive issues work or how many will do the job. But there is one thing for sure: When you are having mood changes and/or cognitive challenges, your body is talking to you, and you should start listening.

When you feel that your mind isn't working as you wish it would, that feeling can take over your life in ways just as serious, acute, and critical as any other disease. In fact, mood changes and cognitive challenges can become medical emergencies because of what they do to your life: They can steal it away from you, and steal you away from your family and your community.

Brain issues might not hurt the way a stomach ulcer hurts. They don't drop you to the floor like a heart attack. They might not be detectable on an X-ray the way osteoarthritis is or on a traditional lab test the way diabetes is. They aren't even necessarily recognized as whole-body issues, even though brain cell function affects every organ, tissue, gland, and secreted hormone in the body. Yet imbalances can impact your life as dramatically as any chronic disease. If you experience anxiety, depression, chronic distraction, concentration issues, or brain fog, or if you have a learning problem, you might receive a formal medical diagnosis like anxiety disorder, or clinical depression, or attention deficit disorder, or attention deficit hyperactivity disorder, or dyslexia—or you might even be told you have an autoimmune disease. You might also get a prescription. What you are less likely to get is a nutrition plan that can smooth out the rough edges and set up your brain chemistry for optimal success.

I have a lot of personal experience with this problem. My daughter, my mother, myself, and many of my clients have been diagnosed with dyslexia or other cognitive difficulties or disabilities, and so I can tell you firsthand the impact that nutrition can have. There are real physical and chemical changes that create these imbalances in the body and there are nutrient-dependent metabolic pathways that affect those balances.

Any therapy that deals with an aspect of brain function must, however, take a multifaceted approach. That's because there are many chemicals that influence brain function that science has defined—chemicals like serotonin, dopamine, epinephrine, and norepinephrine. There are chemicals that we know make us feel good, and whose deficiency we know makes us feel bad. There are brain cell receptor sites throughout the entire body, including, perhaps most significantly, in the gastrointestinal tract. That's good news for anyone seeking to stabilize his or her mood or cognitive symptoms with food.

There is a way through the complexity. If we can support and open pathways for nutrient delivery to the brain so it can be as nourished and as functional as possible, then we can let the body sort the rest out. There are many ways brain dysfunction can happen, but the way we nourish the brain and all its peripheral systems is the same, whether we are attacking chronic clinical depression or helping stabilize attention deficit hyperactivity disorder (ADHD).

Mainstream science is finally beginning to link mood changes and cognitive challenges with measurable physical states in the body, such as: inflammation,[17] elevated cytokinase,[18] and changes in gut bacteria.[19] Mood and cognition can also be influenced by lipid metabolism's causing hormone modulation and immune system dysfunction, not to mention more straightforward-seeming problems like an imbalance in neurochemicals, brain chemistry, and/or hormones. There is also some evidence that clinical depression has a unique metabolic profile and that we may eventually find metabolic markers that can help with a more objective diagnosis and treatment.[20]

It wasn't until I was working with the brilliant Dr. McIntosh at the Brain Recovery Center after a car accident that I learned something: The worse my eczema was, the worse my memory and cognition became. There was a correlation! Dr. McIntosh explained to me that the metabolic pathways that affect autoimmune disorders and inflammation also affect cognition, brain chemistry, and brain function. Thus, brain dysfunction could be both a cause and a symptom of many other chronic issues. One study that got a lot of press suggested that depression is an "allergic reaction" to inflammation in the body.[21] Mood and cognition issues are known side effects of autoimmune disease, and unstable blood sugar is also known to inhibit brain function. So, many kids and adults who are diagnosed with anxiety, depression, and/or focus disorders also have blood sugar issues or compromised immune systems. But if you decide to tackle your mood and/or cognitive issues first, whether or not they are related to hormones, inflammation, or your immune system, a food prescription can help stabilize your situation.

And help is exactly what you need if you are in an acute state of depression or anxiety. You might even need temporary medical intervention. But what about cognitive issues like ADHD or dyslexia? A person diagnosed with dyslexia isn't going to eat his way out of that particular issue, but what he can do is eat in a way that stabilizes the anxiety that goes with it and thereby create the best possible environment to thrive. Someone with concentration or attention issues can benefit from the stability of a nutritional prescription, including the enhanced memory and focus that targeted foods can provide.

Even though these issues affect people in such a wide variety of ways, from learning and communication styles to the ability to form and maintain positive relationships, the goal is always the same: to create homeostasis or balance, stability, and support. The goal is not to numb you or to alleviate any of the cognitive traits or emotions that you have every right to experience, but we do want to establish an internal environment that is nurturing and useful to you. If you do need medication in a crisis, know that I still want to feed you through that crisis because the hope is you won't be in crisis forever, and as you come out of it, you want to have as healthy a body as possible.

THE SELF-DISCOVERY ZONE

If you have mood changes or cognitive challenges, your body is talking to you on a regular basis. Odds are, your friends, family, co-workers, and teachers are talking to you, too. This seems to be the one area of imbalance that people feel comfortable weighing in on, even when they understand virtually nothing about what's going on with you.

But that's no surprise, because most general practitioners don't get much training on mood and cognition, either. Symptoms of mood changes and cognitive challenges can range from subtle to dramatic, and the diagnoses can be elusive. A disturbed circadian rhythm, issues with carbohydrate metabolism, and hormone imbalances can manifest in ways that affect mood and cognition, and some people simply react to a range of stimuli with cognitive dysfunction. I typically see my clients and myself as "multidimensional reactors." For instance, children who are allergic to poison ivy, poison oak, or chlorine in the pool, or who have GI issues like constipation, often began at an early age to manifest cognitive issues as well. As adults, many have positive antinuclear antibody (ANA) titers (a sign of autoimmune dysfunction), imbalances in weight distribution, systemic inflammation such as eczema or rosacea, and many other chronic problems.

This mood and cognition prescription is worth exploring if you experience any of the following symptoms:

- Anxious feelings

- Appetite loss

- Attention problems, or a diagnosis of ADD

- Chemical sensitivity (to chemicals like personal-care products, cleaning products, medications, latex, or chlorine)

- Chronic low levels of pain

- Compulsive behaviors like knuckle cracking, hair twisting, nail biting (or in more extreme cases, cutting and branding)

- Emotional changes: loss of emotions, or excessive emotions

- Fatigue and lethargy after waking in the morning

- Gastrointestinal problems

- Heart palpitations after lying down at night

- Hyperactivity, or a diagnosis of ADHD

- Inability to concentrate on something or pay attention to something for more than a minute or two

- Inability to get a deep, restful sleep

- Insomnia

- Learning disabilities like dyslexia

- Loss of interest in things that used to excite you

- Mania

- Memory loss or uncharacteristic forgetfulness

- Mood swings: feeling extremely happy and then extremely sad

- Numbness and tingling in the hands and feet

- Panic attacks

- Quick to anger or tears

- Ravenous appetite in the evening, after 5:00 p.m.

- Sadness or despair, a pervasive feeling

- Self-medicating with alcohol, food, or drugs to feel calm or interested in things

- Sugar cravings in the afternoon

- Suicidal thoughts

- Tired all the time

- Tremors

DEALING, NOT HEALING

The best way conventional medicine knows to deal with crises that seem behavioral or psychological is through medication, like antidepressants, anti-anxiety medication, antipsychotics, and stimulants; and these medications have saved many lives. Medical intervention can be an important acute-care way to support a body that is in a state of extreme imbalance. We need to support the body that thinks it cannot go on for another moment. We also need to support the body that is having panic attacks or acute anxiety to the extent that it cannot function without sedatives. We need to support the body that cannot focus, cannot live without fear, cannot calm down, or cannot get out of bed. In these emergency situations, medication might be absolutely essential.

But medication is not the end of the story. It cannot be the end because the problem is too important to abandon, even if the primary symptoms are resolved. Depression is not a joke. Panic attacks are not a joke. Suicidal thoughts are not a joke. These are not symptoms of a chronic disorder; they are symptoms of what can become a terminal disease, if not supported. When you have a mood disorder, you *can* die from it. You can also lose everything you need and love because of it. So, we can't take this lightly.

Maybe you've been fired from your job or people you love and need have left you because you can't concentrate, or control your emotions, or use your mind the way you wish you could. Maybe as a kid, your third-grade teacher made you sit on your hands for the entire class because you "wouldn't sit still," and that demoralizing event haunts you to this day. These are serious consequences. You would not get fired because you had heart disease or were experiencing symptoms of diabetes. Maybe social anxiety kept you from attending college or memory or cognition concerns are preventing you from being active in your community. Most people won't leave a spouse because of high cholesterol, but bi-polar disorder? ADHD? It happens all the time.

While medications help, and it's no wonder doctors rush to prescribe them, they don't solve the problems. They mask them. What caused the underlying imbalance? What is underneath the symptoms?

In the last decade and a half, there has been a huge increase in the use of medications for treating mood disorders. According to a report by Medco, a pharmacy benefits management company, more than one in five Americans, and one in four women, were on at least one medication to treat a psychological or behavioral disorder in 2010, with the highest use in women ages forty-five and older, and the greatest increase in men ages twenty to forty-four. This is us—our sisters and brothers, our mothers and fathers, our cousins and co-workers and bosses, and best friends. It's the shopkeeper and the lawyer, the bus driver and the restaurant manager—even the surgeon. Yet, medication to manipulate different metabolic pathways (M) without an eating (E) prescription will not lead to true health.

Treatment of mood disorders and cognitive challenges has come a long way, and it continues to evolve. Once, it was thought that mood disorders were "all in your head" and could not be treated with medication. These were the days of oppressive bed-rest treatments for "hysteria" and commitment to asylums for everything from depression to schizophrenia to epilepsy. It's so funny to me—and I'm sure to other fellow dyslexics such as Charles Schwab, Cher, Ben Foss, and Albert Einstein—that people used to believe dyslexics were "just stupid." Now, we understand that there is a metabolic basis for many of these issues, and this progress has transformed the treatment of mood changes and cognitive challenges into something much more humane.

What happened with this realization, though, was that medication became the be-all and end-all of therapy. Doctors began to give their patients medication as the only treatment, without looking at other aspects of a person's life. A loved one just died? Here's a medication. You lost your job? Here's medication. Don't like yourself? Here's medication. Can't focus? Here's medication.

Fortunately, this is changing, too. Although many psychiatrists still default to medication as the primary treatment for mood disorders, often but not always out of necessity, more doctors are also prescribing talk therapy, EMDR, neural therapy, touch therapy, or other treatments that help the patient deal with problems that could have triggered the imbalance. This can include exploring the source of that depression or anxiety, offering lifestyle organizational strategies for people with concentration issues, and employing tools like meditation or exercise for improving mood and clearing brain fog. We are even seeing occupational therapy prescriptions for children and adults dealing with ADD and ADHD. Hooray! These are all steps in the right direction, and they reflect a more holistic approach to these problems, but we are still missing a huge piece of the puzzle.

We aren't yet seeing food prescriptions coming from doctors. And yet, stimulants to treat attention and hyperactivity disorders (and more recently, binge-eating disorders), selective serotonin uptake inhibitors to treat depression, sedatives to treat anxiety, and many other similar drugs are altering patients' metabolic pathways. If a drug relieves a psychotropic symptom, it does so by manipulating a neurotransmitter manufactured by fat metabolism. Drug companies understand the metabolism very well; they make it their business. But, *every single metabolic pathway altered by a medication designed to treat a mood or cognition issue is nutrient dependent and can be strongly influenced by the right micronutrients.* Rather than treat this huge range of cognitive and mood manifestations, why not get to the root of the problem? Why not create homeostasis in the brain chemistry by stabilizing the metabolic pathways that feed the brain?

By establishing stability, it is possible to define what kinds of interventions will be meaningful. I'm not saying a person shouldn't take an ADHD medication or an antidepressant. What I'm saying is that a stable system, with open and functioning metabolic pathways, will be able to use a prescribed drug in the most efficient way, with the least quantities, without disrupting other pathways or causing disturbing side effects. You are a dynamic, biodiverse human being, and your brain cannot be reduced to an easy fix. But it can be set on the right path and achieve homeostasis, which can put you in the best possible position to live your life successfully.

So, as mentioned earlier, a physician needs to intervene with meds in a crisis situation, but once the person is stabilized, we look at who that person is, where they are, what they are doing—we get the whole picture. Particularly when you are suffering from a mood disorder, it is essential to maintain an adequate supply of amino acids. It is also crucial to support the liver and adrenals. When you consume carbohydrates, you need to be able to metabolize them so you can receive their mood-elevating effects.

Have you ever noticed how your mood changes if you go on a diet or decide to eat better? People often talk about a change in their psyche as a bonus to losing weight or changing their diets. They might say, "Wow, now that I'm eating better, I sleep better! It's so weird!" Trust me, it's not weird. This is not some mysterious side effect. Indeed, I have seen the right nutrition plan allow many people to eventually come off antidepressants, or at minimum to lower their dosage. I've seen people on antianxiety medication that wasn't working

What you eat has a profound effect on your mood. Science now recognizes that adrenal hormones such as cortisol and pancreatic hormones such as insulin affect neurotransmitter balance. Neurotransmitters are not isolated to the brain. For example, serotonin is a very powerful neurotransmitter in the blood that regulates mood balance. And although you might reasonably assume that most of your serotonin is produced in your brain, 95 percent of the serotonin in your body comes from the gut, manufactured by some of the 100 trillion microbes that live in your GI tract. (This is why the gut is sometimes called "the second brain.") Everything you eat impacts the balance of gut microbes and the functioning of the neurotransmitters all along your digestive tract. In fact, your digestive tract contains about 100 million neurons, too, which outnumber all the neurons in your spinal cord. We all accept the fact that food affects the gut, and now we know the gut affects the brain. Therefore, we now know without a doubt that food affects the brain.

well finally get their good effects by changing the foods they were eating. I want you to receive all the benefits and promises the pharmaceutical companies make, but to do that, you might need a little help. These drugs manipulate the way the body uses micronutrients, hormones, and amino acids. But where do the micronutrients, hormones, and amino acids come from? They come from food, of course.

TARGETED PATHWAYS FOR REPAIR

There are thousands of pathways that affect mood, memory, cognition, and focus, which have already been defined by scientists. I can only imagine what is yet to be discovered. But there are a few target areas I love to focus on when we begin to establish a positive homeostasis with mood and cognitive challenges. The goal is to create an environment of stability, in which someone with mood changes or cognitive challenges cannot just survive but also thrive. To do this, we target several crucial pathways:

People often struggle with the inability to concentrate on something for very long, and there is a recent trend to criticize multitasking. Concentration issues can definitely be a matter of a neurochemical imbalance, but in some people, they are a natural trait that once offered an evolutionary advantage. Imagine that you lived in ancient times and you had to build a fire pit for your village. You are working hard, but suddenly a pack of wolves appears from out of the forest. If you don't stop building that fire pit, that's it for you—you will get eaten. So, you need to be able to be aware of more than one thing in your environment, and be able to quickly switch tasks when necessary. Some people also theorize that most of the major inventions and progress in the world have come from those people driven by what we now label as "hyperactivity" and "attention deficits." These people are the dreamers, the ones able to achieve what others thought was impossible.

Unfortunately for many kids, this kind of broad awareness and easy distractibility is not an advantage in the classroom. Kids are expected to sit still at a desk and listen and focus for long periods of time; those who aren't good at this often get labeled as "problems." This societal pressure, rather than the distractibility itself, can contribute to anxiety, causing biochemical changes in the brain due to stress, which can worsen the problem. Anxiety hormones can gum up the receptors for the feel-good hormones, and before long these children are caught in a downward spiral of what feels like failure, anxiety, and eventually depression. It can be very hard to climb back up. It's too bad we don't give distractible kids—and adults, too, because some people never outgrow this trait—an environment in which their natural multitasking and hyperawareness traits could be beneficial, even appreciated. It's fun to imagine such environments on a wider scale: individualized learning in schools, work environments that permit frequent movement or more flexible hours, jobs that can be done from home, and a society in awe of a wider variety of learning styles for all ages.

This is all especially relevant to me because I am an adult who grew up with ADHD and dyslexia; the only reason I'm able to write this book is that my mother created a home environment that allowed me to flourish instead of flounder. My mother often repeated a favorite quote to me: "Everybody is a genius. But if you judge a fish by its ability to climb a tree, it will live its whole life believing that it is stupid." This has carried me through many hard times, when I thought I couldn't do something and must be stupid. She taught me that I had great skills and I could use them to thrive. She also gave me tons of freedom, and although we didn't have a lot of money and lived in a city, my mom made sure my passions were fed: We had a horse, pigs, cattle, and sheep. I was allowed to ride my bike all by myself, all the way out to where we kept our horse. I didn't have the privilege of growing up in Montana or Colorado, but she made me feel normal for having pigs while I was growing up in Southern California. All was always okay. I never felt I should have been or should try to be anything different from what I was. She was a huge advocate for me. I can't tell you how many times I saw her marching down the school hallway as I sat in the office in trouble, and I thought to myself, *Ooh, they are going to be in so much trouble.* My mother always told me that I had a good heart, and that I was meant to use all my energy to help people. And you know what? I really believed her. Now it's my turn. When my own daughter was forced by a teacher to sit on her hands for forty-five minutes to keep her still, I marched right down the hallway just as my own mother had, and I pulled her out of that school and told her she would never have to go there again.

But even if you missed the opportunity window for your child, or you didn't have a free environment growing up, it is never too late for a "happy-ever-after," no matter what your challenges. If you have a difficult time concentrating, create an environment that makes concentration easier. If you have a ton of energy, don't feel forced to come down to "the norm." Elevate the environment to match the energy.

When your environment doesn't match how you feel inside, you can experience anxiety. When you feel the normal rhythm of life isn't going to support you—as if you are dancing and somebody keeps changing the beat or everyone is telling you to sit down and stop it and sit on your hands—it can be hard to remember that it is okay to be who you are.

Create your new environment today. Find the tools to help yourself. Consider occupational therapy, whose proponents are continually discovering amazing technological resources for people with cognitive challenges like ADHD and dyslexia. Stay curious, keep learning, find out what's out there to help you, and continue to craft an environment, and even a career, that uses your strengths. Everyone has those strengths, but if you have been led to believe you don't, then you've been misled. Find your genius, believe my mother's brilliant quote—and if you are truly a fish, stop trying to climb trees and instead swim, swim, swim!

1. **Lipid metabolism,** at the point where fats are being converted to master hormones, which can then be converted to brain and sex hormones. When this pathway isn't working correctly, it creates a disruption in brain chemistry that can manifest in many ways. This is one reason mood changes are so commonly linked to hormonal imbalance.

2. **The adrenal hormones,** which are designed to control adaptation. When the adrenals become inhibited in their action, this subsequently inhibits mood modulation, so we target the adrenals with the micronutrients that support them.

3. **Neurotransmitter receptor sites,** which, when they are impaired, prevent the body from benefiting from neurosteroid, neurotransmitter, and hormone production. No matter what substances your body makes, they won't help you if you can't use them, so we wash and clear out these receptor sites to take full advantage of what your body is producing via fat metabolism.

4. **Gut microbiome,** because although the gut isn't exactly a metabolic pathway, or tied to a specific metabolic pathway, it is a mode of delivery of micronutrients that affects every metabolic pathway. The gut is also loaded with neural tissue. Often considered the second brain, it is important that we feed the body in a way that creates a healthy flora for nutrient transformation in the intestines, as well as for absorption and receptor site activity, thereby maximizing serotonin production and communications between the central nervous system and the gut.

REMOVE, REPAIR, AND RESTORE

To give your body what it needs to stabilize and to nourish neurotransmission, remove mood disorder triggers, negotiate cognitive imbalances, and replenish beneficial gut bacteria, we employ strategic foods that boost mood, improve brain function, and nourish the metabolic pathways the brain utilizes. Specifically, we will:

1. Remove triggers for mood disorders and cognitive imbalance, neurosuppression, and neurostimulation, and organize meals in a way that stimulates micronutrient uptake in the gut.

2. Repair liver function, GI production of neurotransmitters, imbalances between neurosuppression and neurostimulation, and metabolic pathways for neurotransmitter production.

3. Restore the body's natural rhythms through homeostasis in adrenal activity and lifestyle modifications targeted to mood and cognitive balance.

GUIDELINES FOR YOUR MOOD AND COGNITION REPAIR RX

To get the most from your Mood and Cognition Repair prescription, follow these guidelines:

- You will be taking this prescription six times a day for the first five days of each week (by eating six times every day for five days in a row), and then you will be taking this prescription five times a day for the remaining two days of each week. That means you will have three strategic mood-balancing meals every day during the week, plus three targeted mood-balancing snacks for the first five days and two targeted mood-balancing snacks for the last two days of each week. You will take your prescription (eat) every three to four hours, and you will split each week into two parts, eating according to one meal plan for five consecutive days and then another meal plan for the next two consecutive days. Then you repeat the pattern.

- Because in this chapter I attempt to provide support for individuals who are dealing with situational mood fluctuations or mood or cognitive issues that are a disability, the length of application of this prescription can vary drastically. Minimally, I like to see individuals apply this prescription for three months. However, many kids I began working with at an early age who struggled with ADHD have been eating this way for twenty years now. This does not mean you are chained to this way of eating. Rather, it is an incredible support for your brain. Many of my clients notice a definite mood stabilization during the first month, but for long-term stability, give yourself at least three months on this brain-boosting plan. If you object to any of the foods for any reason, just replace them with a different food from the Top 20 Power Foods list or the Foundational Foods List. For example, you could substitute broccoli for lima beans or turkey for mackerel.

- Explain to your doctor not only that you are having mood issues but also that you are working on them with diet. And don't be afraid to say something. People are sometimes afraid to bring up their mood issues to a doctor, not wanting to admit they are depressed or anxious or having panic attacks, or that they aren't doing well at work or in school because of concentration, attention, or learning issues. Yet, this is important information for your doctor and can help justify certain lab tests that can be illuminating. The labs I recommend at the end of this

CULTURED/FERMENTED VEGETABLES

Cultured or fermented (these words are synonymous) vegetables are excellent for promoting a healthy microbiome, and we know that a healthy microbiome influences not just digestion but also mood because 95 percent of the serotonin in your body is manufactured in your gut, much of it by those gut bacteria. This happens because the fermentation process creates enzymes that feed and introduce additional healthy bacteria to the gut.

Examples of cultured vegetables are sauerkraut, kimchi, and pickles; kombucha is a fermented beverage. I recommend trying different brands and different products on a rotating basis, to find those you like but also to add different strains of bacteria to your body. The more diverse your microbiome, the healthier you will be. You can also make your own cultured vegetables at home. You'll find my recipe for fermented salsa on page 190.

chapter can give you and your doctor a more specific idea of where your chemistry might be going out of balance. Put your request in writing with a list of your symptoms.

EAT YOUR MEDICINE: YOUR MOOD AND COGNITION REPAIR RX

The following power foods are excellent for mood balancing, so use them as often as you can, fitting them into your meal maps and then layering them with the items from the Foundational Foods List to fill out your meals. This will add power and speed to your brain-balancing prescription.

This prescription has two parts. You will see two different meal maps here—the first is to be followed for five days of each week, the second meal map is for the last two days of each week. This is easy to remember if you do the first part on Monday through Friday, and the second on the weekend.

My strategy for the first five days on this plan is to create a consistent rate of natural sugar delivery through fruits and healthy fats for their mood-boosting effects, while enhancing cholesterol metabolism. Also we'll infuse your body with healthy fats and proteins to slow the uptake of sugar into your cells. Fats combined with vegetable-based fiber will trigger pregnenolone production, which goes up into the brain tissue after being activated by

TOP 20 POWER FOODS FOR MOOD AND COGNITION	
Apricots	Mackerel
Beef liver (organic only)	Oranges
Broccoli	Oysters
Cantaloupe	Peaches
Carrots	Pumpkin
Cashews	Salmon
Chickpeas	Sardines
Collard greens	Spinach
Cultured (fermented) veggies	Turkey
Lima beans	Walnuts

the adrenals. This has a calming effect on the adrenals and is quick to quell production of crisis hormones.

MEAL MAP FOR MOOD AND COGNITION REPAIR, DAYS 1–5

BREAKFAST	SNACK	LUNCH	SNACK	DINNER	SNACK
Fruit (high or low G.I.) Protein Healthy Fat	Fruit (high or low G.I.) Healthy Fat	Protein Vegetable Complex Carb	Fruit (high or low G.I.) Healthy Fat	Protein Vegetable Complex Carb	Healthy Fat

During the final two days of the week, my strategy is to create foods that are very easy on the GI tract. That's why we move to cooked vegetables, which soften the fiber, while we re-inoculate the gut with the probiotics in cultured vegetables, which contain both pre- and probiotics. This improves the functionality of the microbiome, boosting natural serotonin production and improving communication between the neural tissue in the gut and the central nervous system. Note that for lunch and dinner, you will have two vegetable servings—one of your choice and one cultured.

MEAL MAP FOR MOOD AND COGNITION REPAIR, DAYS 6–7

BREAKFAST	SNACK	LUNCH	SNACK	DINNER	SNACK
Fruit (high or low G.I.) Healthy Fat Vegetable	Vegetable (cooked)	Protein Vegetable (any) Complex Carb Vegetable (cultured)	Vegetable (cooked)	Protein Vegetable (any) Complex Carb Vegetable (cultured)	None

A DAY IN THE LIFE OF MOOD AND COGNITION REPAIR

Here is an example of how you might use the Mood and Cognition Repair power foods and items on the Foundational Foods List to create your own meal plan. Remember to focus on the power foods but add the foundational foods you like and enjoy, too. This is just one way you might put together your meal map; I've included the meal recipes that go with this sample day afterwards (recipe titles appear in boldface in the meal map).

BREAKFAST	SNACK	LUNCH	SNACK	DINNER	SNACK
Citrus Salad	Cantaloupe and cashews	**Slow Cooker Turkey Chili**	Apricots and walnuts	**Dumpling and Turkey Stew**	Olives

RECIPES

CITRUS SALAD

Serves 2

>4 large eggs
>1 tablespoon Dijon mustard
>4 tablespoons orange juice
>4 tablespoons lime juice
>2 tablespoons olive oil
>1/4 teaspoon sea salt
>3/4 teaspoon black pepper
>2 grapefruits
>1 avocado, diced

Place the eggs in a small saucepan and fill with water. Cover and bring the water to a boil over high heat. Turn off the heat and let sit for 10 minutes.

In a mixing bowl, whisk together the Dijon mustard, orange juice, lime juice, olive oil, salt, and pepper.

Segment the grapefruit by peeling and slicing between the white pith. Mix the avocado and grapefruit in a bowl and drizzle with the dressing; toss to coat well.

Peel the boiled eggs and slice or quarter them. Place them on top of the avocado grapefruit mixture, and serve.

SLOW COOKER TURKEY CHILI

Serves 6

>1 pound ground turkey
>2 carrots, diced
>2 celery ribs, diced
>1 15-ounce can diced tomatoes
>1 15-ounce can kidney beans
>1 15-ounce can black beans

3 tablespoons tomato paste

$^3/_4$ cup diced yellow onion

$^1/_2$ cup diced green bell pepper

2 tablespoons chili powder

$^1/_2$ tablespoon turmeric

$^1/_2$ tablespoon garlic powder

$^1/_2$ teaspoon red pepper flakes

$^1/_4$ teaspoon sea salt

$^1/_4$ teaspoon black pepper

In a skillet over medium heat, brown the turkey with a little water until no longer pink, about 5 minutes. Add the turkey and all remaining ingredients to a slow cooker and set on low. Cook for 6 to 8 hours.

DUMPLING AND TURKEY STEW

Serves 8

FOR THE DUMPLINGS

2 cups raw almond flour

1 teaspoon sea salt

$^1/_4$ teaspoon black pepper

2 large eggs

Celery leaves from 3 ribs, chopped (reserve stalks for stew)

FOR THE STEW

5 pounds turkey breast, bone-in

5 quarts vegetable stock

2 carrots, chopped

3 celery ribs, chopped

1 head of broccoli, trimmed and cut into florets

1 small yellow onion, sliced

6 parsley sprigs

6 thyme sprigs

2 rosemary sprigs

2 dried bay leaves

1 teaspoon sea salt

$^1/_2$ teaspoon black pepper

Chopped fresh chives, for garnish

Make the dumplings: In a mixing bowl, combine the flour, salt, pepper, eggs, and celery leaves. Form into balls 1½ tablespoons in size. Cover and refrigerate until ready to use.

Make the stew: Add all the ingredients to a slow cooker and cook on low for 6 to 8 hours. During the last 20 minutes, remove the turkey breast. Pull the meat off the bone and shred it using two forks, then discard the bone and place the meat back in the cooker to finish cooking.

Place the dumplings into the slow cooker on top of the stew. Cook for 20 more minutes.

To serve, spoon a couple dumplings and some stew into each bowl. Garnish with chives, if desired.

SNACK IDEAS FOR MOOD AND COGNITION REPAIR, DAYS 1–5

MORNING AND AFTERNOON SNACKS

For the first two snacks of your day, choose a fruit and a healthy fat, such as:

- Oranges and cashews
- Pumpkin puree mixed with cinnamon and walnuts
- Pear slices with almond butter

EVENING SNACK

As the meal map states, this snack should contain only a healthy fat.

- Raw cashews
- Avocado with sea salt and black pepper
- Raw almonds

Now for a sample of how you can eat during the last two days of the week:

SAMPLE DAY FOR MOOD AND COGNITION, DAYS 6–7

BREAKFAST	SNACK	LUNCH	SNACK	DINNER
Peach-Kale Smoothie	Cooked broccoli	Vegetarian Bean Soup	Cooked kale	Kimchi Salmon Patties

RECIPES

PEACH-KALE SMOOTHIE

Serves 1

- $1/4$ avocado
- 1 cup fresh or frozen peaches
- $3/4$ cup almond milk
- $1/2$ cup fresh kale
- $1/2$ cup ice cubes
- $1/4$ teaspoon stevia (optional)
- Pinch of ground cinnamon (optional)

Combine all the ingredients except the cinnamon in a blender, and blend until smooth, about 1 minute. Top with a sprinkling of the cinnamon.

VEGETARIAN BEAN SOUP

Serves 4

- 6 dried shiitake mushrooms
- 4 cups hot water
- 1 15-ounce can adzuki beans
- $2/3$ cup sauerkraut
- 1 cup uncooked quinoa
- 1 cup thinly sliced yellow onion
- 3 garlic cloves, minced
- 2 teaspoons paprika
- 1 tablespoon tamari
- 6 tablespoons chopped fresh parsley
- $1/4$ teaspoon sea salt
- $1/4$ teaspoon black pepper

Soak the mushrooms in 1 cup hot water for 20 minutes, or until softened. Drain and save the soaking water. Discard the stems and slice the mushroom caps.

Puree the beans in a blender or food processor and set aside.

In a large saucepan or soup pot, combine the remaining water, the mushrooms and soaking liquid, the sauerkraut, quinoa, onion, and garlic. Cook for 30 minutes over low heat.

Add the paprika, tamari, pureed beans, 3 tablespoons of the parsley, and the salt and black pepper to the pot. Simmer for 5 to 10 minutes. Divide among serving bowls and garnish each serving with the remaining parsley.

KIMCHI SALMON PATTIES
Serves 2

FOR THE QUICK PICKLED VEGGIES
1/4 cup thinly sliced carrot

1/4 cup thinly sliced cucumber

1/2 cup thinly sliced green cabbage

3 radishes, trimmed and thinly sliced

1 teaspoon sea salt

2 tablespoons rice vinegar

1 tablespoon stevia

1/8 teaspoon black pepper

FOR THE SALMON CAKES
2 1/2 tablespoons quick-cooking oats

1 large egg

12 ounces skinless salmon fillets

1/2 cup purchased kimchi

1/4 teaspoon black pepper

4 butter lettuce leaves

1 teaspoon Korean red pepper paste or Tabasco, or to taste

2 lemon wedges

Make the pickled veggies: Place the carrot, cucumber, cabbage, and radish in a small bowl. Sprinkle with the salt and use your fingers to rub the salt into the vegetables. In a separate mixing bowl, stir together the rice vinegar, stevia, and pepper to make a quick vinaigrette. Toss the vegetables with the vinaigrette and place in the refrigerator to marinate for about 15 minutes.

To make the salmon cakes, lightly beat the egg and soak the oatmeal in it for 15 minutes.

Peel or carefully slice the skin off the salmon fillets, then place the salmon and kimchi in a food processor and process until smooth. Brush down the sides of the processor with a spoon, then add the beaten egg and the oats. Process just until well incorporated and the salmon mixture holds together.

Make 2 large or 4 small patties by rolling a portion of salmon mixture into a ball and then flattening the ball into a disk about 1/2 inch thick. Refrigerate for 15 minutes (or freeze for future use).

Preheat the oven to 425°F.

Remove the pickled veggies from the refrigerator and squeeze to remove as much excess water as possible. Taste and adjust the seasoning. Set aside.

Place the salmon cakes in a baking dish and bake for 10 to 15 minutes, or until the internal temperature reaches 160°F.

To serve, place 1 or 2 salmon patties (depending on whether you made 2 or 4) atop 2 pieces of lettuce, top with some of the pickled veggies, season with additional salt and pepper to taste. Serve with the lemon wedges.

BONUS: HAYLIE'S FERMENTED SALSA

This bonus recipe is a favorite of mine, so easy to make and so handy to have around when you are trying to incorporate more fermented foods into your diet. The next time you want salsa, start a few days ahead and make this one. Your gut and your brain will thank you.

Makes about 2 quarts

3 pounds ripe tomatoes, chopped
1 medium red onion, chopped
2 jalapeño chiles, minced
1 cup chopped fresh cilantro
4 garlic cloves, minced
Juice of 2 limes
1 1/2 tablespoons sea salt
2 teaspoons ground cumin

Combine the ingredients in a large bowl, then transfer to clean glass jars (leave some room at the top) and screw the lids on tightly. Leave the salsa on the counter for 2 to 3 days, and then refrigerate until ready to use. The flavor will continue to intensify in the fridge.

NOTE: Use this salsa as a topping for meats or veggies, or simply eat it on its own, as a Cultured Vegetable serving. (I know tomatoes are considered a fruit in this book, but when they are cultured in this recipe, they become a Cultured Vegetable.)

RESTORE MOOD BALANCE: TOP THREE NON-FOOD STRATEGIES

- **Cardio, cardio, cardio.** Of all the kinds of exercise you can do, cardio is the best stress reliever. Don't do it so much or so often or so hard, though, that you are hurting yourself. But the fact is that when there is a tiger on your tail, you run—and that burns the anxiety hormones. It's also vasodilating, which helps increase blood flow to the brain.

- **Talk therapy or occupational therapy.** I'm dividing this one into two categories, depending on whether your mood changes are situational or long-term cognitive challenges. For those with situational depression, relationship problems, career issues, or other temporary situations that make one feel depressed, anxious, or unable to cope, talk therapy can be a huge help, and I highly recommend it. For those with biochemical or long-term cognitive challenges, talk therapy might be less useful. Occupational therapy, on the other hand, can help those with long-term problems to access skills and tools in their environment. Especially for memory, concentration, and learning issues, occupational therapy can help people find organizational tools, like the Livescribe Pen, software programs, computer audible programs, special fonts for dyslexia, and other ways to navigate the environment for greater success. This goes for things like clinical depression, too. If that's your issue, you need to know how to recognize your triggers and prepare yourself by creating a supportive environment. This is crucial. When you watch the weather report and you see that it's going to be a doomy-gloomy day, occupational therapy can help you know what to do to prepare for it.

I often recommend that clients find an occupational therapist who works with neurologists who handle brain injuries, because those neurologists grasp the nature of depression and anxiety and cognitive fatigue better than others. These neurologists also know the occupational therapists who are experts at creating the right environment for dealing with these issues. There are multiple resources available for people who need a little cognitive boost. Get the help that's out there!

- **Organize.** For mood changes like depression and anxiety that are not emergencies, one of the best (and possibly the most boring, but in this case that is a good thing) strategies is to do non-emotion-based organizational tasks. The more complex or occupying, the better. Do things that involve numbers, or sorting, or cleaning, or a lot of back-and-forth carrying. These activities help stabilize mood and occupy the brain, and can sometimes break the wave of a mood change to reorient you so you feel calmer and more in control. Of course, this is never enough on its own, but it can be an effective intervention at a moment of sadness or nervousness.

BRIEFING YOUR DREAM TEAM

This is a tricky one, because there are basically zero markers for mood imbalances and cognitive challenges. That is why it is so easy to misdiagnose those conditions. Is that ADHD really an anxiety disorder? Is that brain fog really a symptom of autoimmunity? Is that depression situational or biochemical? For these reasons, I recommend a pretty broad swath of lab tests, which helps draw the big picture and point to where the imbalances might be. I recommend asking your doctor for these tests if you are struggling with mood issues and/or cognitive challenges:

- **ANA titers:** Antinuclear antibodies are substances produced by the immune system that attack the body's own tissues. This test helps detect autoimmune disorders, or can help narrow down unexplained symptoms such as arthritis, rashes, or chest pain. ANA is reported as a "titer" (this just means the concentration as determined by a laboratory process called titration) and high titers suggest the possibility of an autoimmune condition (low to nonexistent titers are normal). Mood changes and cognitive challenges can be a precursor to autoimmune issues, so it's good to know if yours are a symptom of autoimmunity.

- **Sed rates, or erythrocyte sedimentation rate (ESR):** This test reveals inflammatory activity in your body that can lead to mood changes and even cognitive dysfunction. It can help diagnose and monitor inflammatory diseases like rheumatoid arthritis.

- **Thyroid tests:** You have to go beyond the traditional panel. When people start to have low energy, depression, or anxiety, thyroid issues can be a cause. For example, in Hashimoto's thyroiditis, anxiety can get extremely serious. Again, these tests help us to understand the pathways and can guide treatment. If your ANA titer (see above) turns out to be positive, see Chapter 11 and ask for these particular thyroid tests:

  - *TSH, or thyroid stimulating hormone.* This shows how hard the pituitary is working to communicate with your thyroid. The test is a good one to run if you are experiencing fatigue, exhaustion, and brain fog.

  - *T4.* Your thyroid gland produces T4, and abnormal levels can also be related to fatigue. If T4 is below normal, ask your doctor about hypothyroidism.

  - *T3.* Your liver converts T4 into T3 to make it bioavailable, and this hormone has a major impact on your metabolism. Low levels of T3 are often associated with a disrupted circadian rhythm, weight gain, and depression.

- *Reverse T3 (RT3).* Many doctors aren't used to running this test, but ask for it because these misshapen thyroid hormones block T3 receptor sites and could be the cause of low T3. Reverse T3 could be associated with stubborn excess weight and possibly with autoimmune disease. If your RT3 is high, avoid soy foods and be even more diligent about getting enough sleep.

- *TgAB or anti-thyroid antibody (ATA).* Abnormal amounts of these thyroid antibodies could be preventing you from utilizing thyroid hormones. This can be associated with fatigue, chronic low-grade infection symptoms (like feverish feeling and swollen lymph nodes). If your levels are high, avoid nightshade vegetables (tomatoes, bell peppers, and eggplant), which can aggravate this condition because of their inflammatory effect in some people.

- *Thyroid peroxidase.* This enzyme destroys T4 before it can produce T3. It can manifest as chronic allergies or indicate an autoimmune disorder.

Many functional medicine doctors are going even further, doing urine tests to check for other more transitory indications of mood, such as abnormal levels of:

Epinephrine
Norepinephrine
Cortisol
Serotonin
Dopamine

They are also testing for:

- **PEA, or beta-phenylethylamine:** This is a neurohormone neurotransmitter important for focus and concentration.

- **Toxins:** Toxins can inhibit neurotransmitters and disrupt neurologic and neurotransmitter pathways. If you want to explore this avenue, ask your doctor about tests for the presence of heavy metals, PCBs, volatile solvents, plastics, parabens, organophosphate pesticides, and chlorinated pesticides. It blows my mind that studies are done on animals before a drug is approved, yet chemicals that are supposed to kill animals aren't supposed to hurt us. It's bizarre.

Note: If you benefit from an SSRI (selective serotonin reuptake inhibitor, commonly prescribed for depression and/or anxiety) but are having difficulty with some of the side effects, ask your doctor about having your serotonin compounded naturally. You can do this with other hormones, too. I've seen a lot of people benefit clinically from doing so.

SOMETHING TO CHEW ON

When my clients are dealing with mood and cognition issues, I encourage them to be open about it. It's okay to stop and say, "Hey, I'm confused." In fact, it's one of the most empowering statements that a neurologist taught me: "Hold on a minute, I'm confused."

Being able to announce this confusion released my anxiety about my brain injury rehab. If you are feeling anxious or depressed or confused, or just completely baffled about what someone is saying, or what is happening, or what you are supposed to do, it's perfectly all right to say so. You can also say that you have a problem, such as "I'm dyslexic," or "I have ADHD," or "I'm feeling a little anxious right now." You're not labeling yourself—you're making yourself feel better. It quells the anxiety, whereas anxiety just makes everything you're trying to deal with so much worse. So own it, say it, and use the power. There is no shame in your game!

PART FOUR

Your Body Is Screaming

CHAPTER 10

Metabolic Syndrome, Blood Sugar Issues, Prediabetes, and Diabetes

As we begin to see disease manifest—chronic, multifaceted issues with complex symptom profiles and tendencies to progress to multiple layers of disease processes—it's no wonder the body is screaming for help. But it is never too late to listen, to calm those screams, first to a dull roar and then to an "outside voice" perhaps—and maybe, eventually, to a civil conversation, a whisper, and . . . quiet. When the body starts screaming, things get more involved, but even so, many chronic conditions can be reversed or successfully managed so as to have a healthy dialogue in the body.

One of the most common and complex and frustrating of these conditions is diabetes. Diabetes gives us plenty of warning, and it is hardly rare. According to the Centers for Disease Control, 9.3 percent of the U.S. population had diabetes in 2014. That's 29.1 million people—and there are an estimated 27.8 percent more who have not been diagnosed. Prediabetic conditions are likely even more common. According to the American Diabetes Association, in 2012, 86 million Americans age twenty or older had prediabetes. Geez, that sounds like practically everybody!

Diabetes and its precursor conditions, which fall under a host of names like prediabetes (which is sometimes called the metabolic syndrome, syndrome X, or insulin resistance), and closely related conditions like polycystic ovarian syndrome (PCOS) are a huge, huge problem. (PCOS is a disorder in blood sugar, unstable production of insulin or insulin resistance, and disruption of the balance between sex and blood sugar hormones.) If you have any of these conditions—diabetes or a condition that foreshadows it—your body has been whispering and talking to you about it for a very long time. Now that talk has turned into a scream. Did you hear anything it was trying to tell you? There had to be some digestion hints, some inability to convert food to micronutrients, especially carbohydrates (as discussed in Chapter 5). There had to have been some difficulty converting sugar to energy (as mentioned in Chapter 6). There had to have been an issue with hormone production or hormone receptor site conversion (as in Chapter 7), because insulin is a hormone. There was likely an issue with lipid metabolism, because lipid metabolism issues are a common red flag that blood sugar issues are on their way, especially when elevated triglycerides are along for the ride. Remember, one of the common side effects of statin use is the onset of type 2 diabetes. And chances are, there were mood changes and cognitive challenges happening, too. In other words, the issues discussed in every chapter of this book up to this point can all end up as diabetes. The conversation has probably been happening in your body for a long time, but until now maybe you haven't received the right prescription for true healing. As a society, we are desperate for this prescription. The good news is that the National Institutes of Health has stated that diabetes is a disorder of the metabolism, and the definition of *metabolism* is "to change." So that's what we're going to do: We are going to change your environment to change the metabolic adaptations your body has made to get you to this point.

The problem is, this is a complex matter, yet modern medicine has to a large extent reduced it to one thing: sugar. Yes, it's true that refined sugars—white sugars—are bad for your health. But what about the healthy sugars we get from complex carbs, fruits, and veggies? Many individuals, metabolically, are having a problem with those sugars, as well. This problem, then, is not caused by those healthful foods. It is caused by a dysfunction in one or more of the metabolic pathways that control sugar metabolism. Those individuals aren't, on a cellular level, realizing the benefits of the sugars they eat; they are starving on a cellular level. If this is you, there is a void in your cells that is screaming out to be filled with fuel in the form of sugar, so you crave the processed kind in an attempt to get sugar into the bloodstream quickly. You *need* sugar.

In Chapter 6, we talked about four ways to get energy. Three of those four ways are completely dependent on sugar metabolism. And energy is crucial;

it's not just for getting through the workday or chasing your kids around. It exists on a cellular level so you can create energy and rebuild your body. We create Essential Energy with the metabolism of carbohydrates into sugar and the conversion of sugar into fuel. We create Crisis Energy with the conversion of sugar into fuel. The Metabolic Energy we create with exercise is the burning of sugar stored in the muscle as glycogen. This is why many individuals dealing with diabetes and prediabetes will have muscle wasting and fatigue—they need Metabolic Energy but they can't store the sugars they need to create it.

I understand why people blame diabetes on the consumption of sugar. There is a direct correlation: As our sugar consumption has skyrocketed, so have our diabetes rates. According to the U.S. Department of Agriculture, the average American consumes about 156 pounds of sugar each year, up from about 20 pounds per year in 1920. Soda is the leading culprit, but candy, desserts, and other processed foods are close behind. But we also know that sugar consumption doesn't always lead to diabetes. All of us can name people who consume copious amounts of sugar and never manifest a blood sugar issue.

When you have blood sugar issues, whether it's prediabetes or full-blown type 2 diabetes, the problem isn't that you eat too much sugar. Just like having high cholesterol isn't because you eat too much fat. Actually, it's the other way around. There is a reason you keep wanting sugar and can't stop eating it. It is because you can't metabolize it. Your body is trying to tell you something with those sugar cravings. You have a blood sugar issue, and you have a blood sugar issue *because* you are not metabolizing sugar. You aren't getting the sugar into your cells and muscles and liver, where it belongs. That sugar, which is so valuable to the proper functioning of your cells, is wandering around outside after curfew, causing trouble. Meanwhile, the cells that need to use sugar for fuel are starving.

What I often tell my clients who have blood sugar issues is that they are, in fact, starving on cellular, structural, and hormonal levels. Sometimes they look at me as if I'm crazy. Possibly it's because some are overweight, so the idea that they could be starving seems unbelievable to them. Yet excess body weight piles on easily in the presence of blood sugar issues and is actually a symptom of that starvation. When you cannot access the fuel that is designed to be delivered to your cells, biochemically you are experiencing famine. That's why you are always hungry. That's why you overeat. You are never satisfied.

To deal with the complex disorder that is diabetes (and all its precursors), we have tended to distill the problem to sugar and insulin, doing a great disservice to our health. In reality, blood sugar issues involve so much more—transport hormones, serotonin, gut bacteria, neurotransmitters, the adrenal response, glucocorticosteroids (created from cholesterol metabolism), adiponectin (secreted from the fat cells), and aldosterone. These affect either the transport or the delivery of sugar into or out of the cells, muscles, and liver. The fact that you are not metabolizing sugar is not as simple as not secreting insulin, or insulin's failing to take sugar into the cell. It's so much more complicated than that.

Diabetes is what many in the medical community consider an end diagnosis, but in reality it is the beginning of, or gateway to, coronary heart disease, Alzheimer's disease, neuropathy, diabetic ulcers, and more. The road doesn't end with diabetes, but it does go downhill from there. As the metabolic pathways become less efficient, the hormone receptor sites become less active; the carrier proteins then become imbalanced, hormone production becomes dysfunctional, and the body begins to create metabolic disorders that foreshadow what's to come. We need to feed metabolic repair and create health. And yes, we can do this!

Your Dynamic Body

As you work your way through this book, you will notice the many crossover symptoms and intersecting metabolic pathways involved. Everything is connected. Your body is one complex, intertwined, and interrelated system. For example, cholesterol affects hormones, which affect mood as well as blood sugar. Blood sugar affects gut bacteria, which affect digestion and mood, and which also affect cholesterol metabolism. This is why a reductionist approach doesn't create health. When I give a prescription for the end disorder, my goal is always to correct the wrong turn made earlier along the road. Where did you go left when you should have gone right? If your primary issue is blood sugar, then the goal is to get you fed on a cellular level. And you may notice that other issues you've had, that existed downstream, will also be resolved.

THE SELF-DISCOVERY ZONE

Maybe you know you have diabetes or prediabetes, or maybe you just suspect it or want to prevent it because you've seen family and friends struggle with it. There are thousands of metabolic pathways that regulate hormone disorders that affect the blood sugar, so you might have many or just a few of these symptoms that indicate a blood sugar imbalance. Depending on your metabolic journey, some or all of these symptoms can manifest:

- Appetite that seems insatiable
- Arm hair that thickens (a classic symptom)
- Bad breath
- Body hair loss, leg hair especially; women will sometimes lose leg hair but gain arm and chin hair
- Carbohydrate cravings that seem excessive
- Confusion or lack of mental clarity
- Abnormal fasting blood sugar
- Abnormal fasting insulin
- Hair growth in women on the face or chest
- Hair loss at the crown in men and women
- Midsection weight gain that feels soft
- Menstrual cycle that becomes irregular
- Muscle development difficulties; it becomes difficult to gain muscle
- Numbness, neuropathy, especially in the hands and feet
- Sugar cravings
- Thirst that is constant and unrelieved by drinking water, and/or higher water consumption than is normal for you
- Tingling in hands and feet
- Elevated triglycerides

- Urination that is more frequent than usual

- Vitamin D deficiency

- Weight gain that seems to be a direct cause of carbohydrate consumption

DEALING, NOT HEALING

The conventional view of blood sugar and insulin issues is pretty straightforward: When you have too much sugar in your blood, your body responds by releasing insulin, which is supposed to shuttle sugar into your cells where it can be used for energy. Typically, this complex issue is distilled down to two things:

1. You are eating too much sugar.

2. You are not producing enough insulin.

When these two conditions are present, for whatever reason, a doctor might address the first by giving some dietary advice: don't eat sugar. The second is typically addressed with medication, as the first line of defense.

Medications that work to regulate blood sugar and insulin levels, or even the injection of insulin itself to keep blood sugar at bay, are common and widely prescribed. Some of them work on insulin, while some of them work to bind sugar and wash it out of the bloodstream. They all, however, work toward the same end: fixing the blood chemistry. Yet this is the end result of blood sugar issues, not the cause. The solutions make sense in an acute situation because if you have too much sugar or insulin in your blood, that's dangerous, even deadly. But why just mop up what's wrong rather than wiping out the real issue? That real issue is, Why aren't you metabolizing sugar?

The answer isn't simple. There are many factors involved beyond just producing insulin and taking sugar into the cells. What else is going on? What is happening in your gut and microbiome? Are your salivary glands triggering insulin secretion when you chew your food? Are your stress hormones nudging you toward insulin resistance? Are you creating the proper hormones through lipid metabolism? Do you have an imbalance in the sex hormones that affect carrier proteins? What about depression or anxiety—has that affected your carbohydrate metabolism? What about the M? What about the "me"? All of these things and more can affect your body's ability to metabolize sugar.

When you develop diabetes, this is what happens:

- The pancreas begins to elevate its secretion of insulin by attempting to modulate sugar in the blood, pulling stress and crisis hormones from the adrenals.

- The body down-regulates the metabolic cycle of energy formation because glucose cannot make its way into the cells to feed this metabolic pathway.

- The body begins to access extra sugars from the smooth muscle of the heart, liver, and muscles, adding additional stress to the functions of cholesterol metabolism, mood modulation, body morphing, and infection defense.

Diabetes is like a leak in the roof, and medications like insulin or metformin are like the bucket you put under the leak. Or maybe not even a bucket—just a sponge. That sponge might soak up some of the water, but it doesn't fix the hole in the roof and it doesn't stop the water from coming in. To address diabetes, then, we need to address sugar metabolism; and to address sugar metabolism, we need to address hormones. Remember—hormones are manufactured from the food we eat, and when and how we eat food determine the level and rate of hormone secretion.

I'm disturbed by the preponderance of "food" being sold as "diabetic," usually right there next to the testing strips. Everything is sugar free, but contains hardly any real food ingredients. These products are all devoid of nutrients, and remember that metabolic pathways are nutrient dependent—and that diabetes is a disorder of the metabolism. Unfortunately, because diabetes is an epidemic, it is also a cash cow for manufacturers. I've even seen ordinary lotions labeled for the diabetic. Rubbing said lotion on your legs will *not* reverse or in any other way affect your diabetes.

If you are on diabetes medication, you desperately need a nutritional protocol designed to stabilize your blood sugar, so you need to get your doctor involved and make sure your diabetic testing and your testing for medication efficacy are synchronized with your eating plan. If your medication isn't keeping your levels stable, all day and every day, your potential for serious side effects, such as neuropathy, cardiovascular disease, and dementia, is even greater. Yet it's common for people with blood sugar and insulin issues to be prescribed medications without also being given a nutrition plan.

Once you start disrupting the balance your body has created with that medication, without also providing the nutrients it needs so it can correct itself and create a new balance, there will be problems and side effects, including severe muscle wasting. Metformin is a difficult medication to come off of, but time and time again I have worked with clients and their doctors to achieve just that. There are huge benefits in establishing the stability that allows you to reduce the medication dose. When you reduce the dose, you gain the ability and potential to reduce the side effects.

WHAT SCIENCE SAYS IS TRUE

Want nine more reasons to heal, not deal? People who have diabetes also tend to have a lot of other health issues, called comorbid conditions. According to the American Diabetes Association, diabetes often occurs in conjunction with:

- Hypoglycemia
- Hypertension
- Dyslipidemia (high LDL blood cholesterol)
- Death from cardiovascular disease
- Hospitalization for heart attack
- Stroke
- Blindness and other eye problems
- Kidney disease
- Amputations

Don't fret. Remember, E + M = H. You can get there with the right prescriptions.

TARGETED PATHWAYS FOR REPAIR

Your body has an amazing ability to heal itself, to make things right again. When you don't foster a stable, nutrient-rich environment, however, your body will have a much harder time healing and repairing the mechanisms that have gone awry. Every day that your blood sugar and insulin remain stable is a day that your body can spend righting the wrongs. Every day that it goes out of control with wild highs and precipitous lows, your body has to fight for its life (meaning *your life*) rather than solving the stickier problems going on at the cellular level. In other words, to encourage healing, you must create stability. I'm not a believer in white-knuckling it, of muscling your way

DON'T FAST! (DON'T EVEN SKIP BREAKFAST!)

If you have a prediabetic condition or diabetes, don't skip meals. Ever. Though many diabetic medications are appetite suppressants, skipping a meal is the worst thing you can do for blood sugar control. Intermittent fasting is trendy these days; the idea is to skip meals here and there, to allow your body a break from digestion so it can heal. This sounds great in theory, but intermittent fasting is one of the worst things you can do to correct a blood sugar issue like diabetes. Think about it: You are already starving at a cellular level. Imagine saying to a starving person, "I'm going to take away your one source of food so you can get *really creative* in how you find nourishment." That would be cruel. We all have different metabolic journeys, and intermittent fasting might work for some people. In fact, fasting might be okay once in a while for those who don't have a metabolic disorder (although I don't ever recommend skipping breakfast). But if you do have a metabolic disorder, then fasting will be encouraging catabolism, which is the body's breaking down of your own structure (bone, hair, skin, nails, muscle) for survival.

The next time you think about skipping breakfast and getting through the morning on your cup of coffee, imagine me in the background, shaking my head and wagging my finger. You are already starving—please don't add insult to injury. Remember, the goal is to create metabolic stability through food, with as little medication intervention as possible.

through, or of denying yourself a complete food group. I want you to heal and bring your body to the best balance possible.

When doctors refer their patients to our clinic, the mutual goal is clear: to create metabolic stability through food and with as little medication intervention as possible. I also have a few additional pathways I seek to repair:

- The production and secretion of enzymes and hormones that regulate blood sugar.

- The production of an adequate supply of carrier proteins to get those enzymes and hormones to their receptor sites.

- The transportation of sugar into the cells with a subsequent efficient conversion of that sugar to energy.

REMOVE, REPAIR, AND RESTORE

I want to get you fed on a cellular level! To do that, we strike a balance in the amount of insulin, sugar, and carrier proteins in the bloodstream, and we attempt to wash the inefficient receptor sites on the cell walls so that sugar can be taken into the cell and converted into energy. For your blood sugar prescription, we are going to concentrate on three things:

1. Remove the refined sugars that inhibit proper enzyme, flora, and hormone production, and any blood sugar instability, by establishing a frequent strategic food intervention.

2. Repair the production and uptake of hormones, enzymes, and flora related to blood sugar stability.

3. Restore a healthy metabolic consumption, storage, and conversion of sugars in the body, including through lifestyle changes that encourage healthy sugar metabolism.

GUIDELINES FOR YOUR BLOOD SUGAR REPAIR RX

To get the most from your blood sugar nutritional prescription, be sure to do the following:

- You will be taking this prescription six times every day (by eating six times every day). That means you will have three strategic blood sugar stabilizing meals and three targeted blood sugar stabilizing snacks each day. You will take your prescription (eat) every three to four hours.

- Typically, my clients stay on this prescription a minimum of three months *after* their chemistry has stabilized. If medication intervention is necessary, some of my clients stay on this prescription for a lifetime. Many diabetics check their blood sugar daily, and you could notice changes in your daily blood sugar values within forty-eight hours, so be sure to partner with your doctor to monitor any reduction needed in medication. Given the complexity of this scream your body is letting out, you may need long-term repair to invoke lifelong results. One of the best markers of your progress is hemoglobin A1C, which is an approximately ninety-day average of blood sugar values. Minimally, hemoglobin A1C should be monitored every ninety days. Once these values are stable, you remain on this prescription for a minimum of another three months . . . or a lifetime.

- If you object to any of the foods for any reason, just replace them with a different food from the Foundational Foods List or the Top 20 Power Foods for Blood Sugar Repair list. For example, you could substitute beef for turkey or olives for raw nuts.

- If you have been diagnosed with diabetes, you may already be on medication. Don't jump off it. Stay closely connected to your doctor and explain that you are working with food therapy so as to improve your condition, then ask for lab tests to continually monitor your blood sugar and insulin so that eating this way begins to stabilize your chemistry, you can adjust your medication accordingly (and, it is hoped, eventually go off it with your doctor's approval). Balance, stability, and consistency are crucial for blood sugar issues, and lab tests can be revealing. If you are currently doing blood sugar testing or consistent testing for insulin, blood sugar, and hemoglobin A1C, this is the time to really make sure you stay on schedule with your doctor, because the goal of this food protocol is to cause a reduction in hemoglobin A1C and to even-out the blood sugar and insulin levels. If you have a diabetes diagnosis, you should already have lab results for some standard tests, but I recommend some additional ones at the end of this chapter for more information. Remember to write down your lab request along with your current symptoms.

- Remember to drink half your body weight in ounces of spring water every day, up to 100 ounces.

EAT YOUR MEDICINE: YOUR BLOOD SUGAR REPAIR RX

My strategy is for you to keep all fruit consumption to before 2:00 p.m. with the exception of eating fruit before workouts. I also want you to add a serving of protein after all workouts. You will have complex carbs at dinner and a healthy fat and protein before bed. The reason for this is that, later in the day, the body is metabolically challenged. With diabetes, especially, the body has difficulty accessing the cells for sugar delivery. Adding a complex carb in the evening feeds the starving cells. Why choose complex carbs instead of fruit? Because fruit and carbs stimulate different enzymes, and carbs work better to stabilize blood sugar in the fat and flora, while fruit does a better job of stabilizing sugar in the pancreas.

Also, using the fat and a protein right before bed pushes a little bit harder on enzyme and hormone production right before sleep. This prevents the body from going after sugar stores in the muscles while it sleeps. One of the ways we see this clinically is by testing the diabetic, especially gestational diabetics (who are more fragile) right before bed and right after waking up. Often we find a higher blood sugar in the morning than before bed, which is not a normal result. It's not because the person is eating while sleeping; it's because the body is scavenging sugar from the muscle.

TOP 20 POWER FOODS FOR BLOOD SUGAR REPAIR

This is your Top 20 Power Foods list. Choose foods from this list whenever you have the opportunity, and supplement these with foods from the Foundational Foods List to round out your meals. These foods will stabilize your blood sugar and insulin and feed the mechanisms of sugar metabolism.

Artichokes

Avocados

Beef (grass-fed)

Bell peppers

Cauliflower

Chia seeds

Coconut milk

Dark leafy greens, especially dandelion greens and spinach

Eggplant

Fresh herbs, especially parsley, rosemary, and chives

Garlic

Green beans

Lettuce

Nuts, raw—all types

Olives

Onions

Turkey (organic)

Vinegar—all types without added sugar

Warming spices like chili powder, cayenne pepper, cinnamon, and turmeric

Zucchini

MEAL MAP FOR BLOOD SUGAR REPAIR, DAYS 1–7

BREAKFAST	SNACK	LUNCH	SNACK	DINNER	SNACK
Complex Carb Protein Healthy Fat	Protein Vegetable	Protein Vegetable Healthy Fat Fruit (low G.I.)	Protein Vegetable	Complex Carb Protein Healthy Fat Vegetable	Protein Healthy Fat (within 1 hour of bed)

A DAY IN THE LIFE OF BLOOD SUGAR REPAIR

Here is an example of how you might fill out your meal map as you work to repair your blood sugar imbalance and the pathways of sugar metabolism. This is a sample day I've employed with my clients, but you can use the meal map to combine foods in the appropriate categories in any way you choose. Recipes follow for the choices shown in boldface type.

SAMPLE DAY FOR BLOOD SUGAR REPAIR, DAYS 1–7

BREAKFAST	SNACK	LUNCH	SNACK	DINNER	SNACK
Breakfast Beef Wrap	Sardines over spinach leaves	**Baked Salmon with Roasted Cauliflower**	Green beans with turkey bacon	**Chicken Marinara Pasta**	Turkey jerky and olives

RECIPES

BREAKFAST BEEF WRAP

Serves 2

> 8 ounces lean ground beef
> 1 tablespoon chili powder
> 1 teaspoon ground cumin
> 2 teaspoons chopped fresh cilantro, divided
> Sea salt
> Freshly ground black pepper
> 2 tablespoons olive oil
> 1/2 small yellow onion, diced
> 1/2 cup water
> 2 sprouted-grain or spelt tortillas
> 1/2 avocado, diced
> Dash of Tabasco (optional)
> 1 tablespoon salsa (optional, see Haylie's Fermented Salsa, page 190)

In a bowl, combine the meat, chili powder, cumin, 1 teaspoon of the cilantro, 1/2 teaspoon salt, and 1/2 teaspoon pepper.

Put the olive oil in a sauté pan over medium heat. Add the onion and cook for

1 minute. Turn the heat to high and add the ground meat mixture and the water, then cook until no longer pink, 5 to 7 minutes.

Heat the tortillas in a separate pan over medium heat just until they are warmed through.

In the center of each tortilla, place half the beef mixture, some of the remaining teaspoon cilantro, half the avocado, the Tabasco, and salt and pepper to taste. Tuck the ends of the tortilla into the center and roll to enclose the filling.

BAKED SALMON WITH ROASTED CAULIFLOWER

Serves 2

  1 head cauliflower, trimmed and cut into florets
  4 tablespoons olive oil, divided
  $1/2$ lemon, cut in half (more if desired)
  $1/4$ teaspoon red pepper flakes
  Sea salt
  Freshly ground black pepper
  2 6-ounce wild-caught salmon fillets
  2 cups trimmed and sliced green beans (in 1-inch pieces)
  $1/2$ small yellow onion, thinly sliced
  2 teaspoons chopped fresh dill

Preheat the oven to 425°F.

In a mixing bowl, combine the cauliflower with 1 tablespoon of the olive oil, a squeeze of $1/4$ lemon, the red pepper flakes, and $1/2$ teaspoon each salt and pepper. Spread the seasoned cauliflower on a baking sheet and roast for 20 to 25 minutes, or until the tops are browned. Use a fork to test for doneness; the tines should easily pierce the cauliflower stems when done.

Meanwhile, rub 1 tablespoon of oil on the salmon and then season with some salt and pepper. Place the fillets skin side down on a nonstick baking sheet or in an ovenproof nonstick pan. Bake until the salmon is cooked through, 12 to 15 minutes.

While the salmon is baking, heat the remaining 2 tablespoons oil in a medium sauté pan over high heat, then stir in the green beans and onion, and lightly season with salt and pepper; heat until beans are tender, about 5 minutes.

Toss the roasted cauliflower with the green beans, then place on serving plates alongside the salmon. Garnish the salmon with the dill and serve with the remaining $1/4$ lemon, cut in half.

CHICKEN MARINARA PASTA

Serves 4

7 tablespoons olive oil

1 small yellow onion, diced

5 garlic cloves, minced

1 28-ounce can diced tomatoes

1 teaspoon dried oregano

1 teaspoon fresh thyme

1/2 teaspoon fresh rosemary

2 teaspoons chopped fresh parsley

2 tablespoons cashews

4 teaspoons nutritional yeast

Sea salt

8 ounces brown rice penne or other tubular pasta

4 4-ounce boneless, skinless chicken breasts

Freshly ground black pepper

16 small to medium basil leaves

Heat 4 tablespoons of the olive oil in a casserole or heavy pot over medium-high heat. Add the onion and garlic, and sauté until the onion is translucent, about 10 minutes. Add the tomatoes and herbs, and reduce the heat to low. Simmer, uncovered, until the sauce thickens somewhat, about 1 hour.

In a food processor, combine the cashews, nutritional yeast, and 1/4 teaspoon salt until a fine powder.

Bring a stockpot half-full with water to a boil over high heat. Add the pasta and cook for 8 to 10 minutes, or as directed on the box. Drain and toss the hot pasta with the marinara sauce.

Season the chicken with some salt and pepper. Heat 2 tablespoons olive oil in a large skillet over high heat. Add the chicken and cook 5 to 7 minutes, turning once, until the internal temperature has reached 165°F.

Serve the pasta on plates with the sautéed chicken on top. Sprinkle the cashew powder evenly across the top, and garnish with basil leaves and the remaining tablespoon of olive oil.

MORNING AND AFTERNOON SNACKS

Remember, choose a protein and a veggie, such as the following:

- Nitrate-free deli roast beef wrapped around raw dandelion leaves or other dark leafy greens
- Ground beef sautéed with chopped bell peppers
- Nitrate-free turkey slices rolled up in romaine leaves
- Celery sticks and cold chicken slices

EVENING SNACK

As the meal map states, this snack should contain only a protein and a healthy fat.

- Turkey bacon and raw almonds
- Steak strips or ground beef mixed with avocado cubes

RESTORE BLOOD SUGAR BALANCE: TOP THREE NON-FOOD STRATEGIES

Your food prescription always comes first, but when you add these lifestyle strategies, your progress will be even more profound. When your body is screaming, it is crucial to do everything you can to get yourself healthy again, and these strategies will make a big difference.

LIFT WEIGHTS

A doctor being interviewed on a morning show recently said something like, "To get rid of belly fat, you have to lift heavy weights." I nodded, interested and excited to hear him explain why—however, he didn't appear to know, he wasn't sure why. Well, I'll tell you why. Belly fat forms as a result of blood sugar metabolism issues—the same ones that can lead to diabetes, which is why belly fat is often an indicator of diabetes or a prediabetic condition. When you have too much sugar circulating in your blood and it can't get into your cells and muscles, you need to give it some help in getting there. Lifting heavy weights results in micro tears in the muscles, and these tears can help open the gates for sugars to enter the muscles. So, always eat fruit before and eat protein after lifting weights, thereby strategically bookending a workout with food.

SLEEP

Get eight to ten hours of deep sleep every night, whenever possible. Sleep is incredibly important for insulin stabilization. Supplements to promote sleep, like melatonin or a seed extract from the *Zizyphus spinosa* plant, can help. Melatonin knocks you out, and *Zizyphus* keeps you out, promoting deep restorative sleep. Make sure you have a dark environment, free of electronics. Dark environments stimulate the pineal gland for deeper sleep; the pineal gland can sense light and doesn't allow you to go into as deep a sleep when there are lights or a television on. And look for things that could be disrupting your sleep, such as sleep apnea or electrolyte imbalances that might bring about restless leg syndrome. Sleep deprivation is known to reduce insulin sensitivity, so adequate sleep is crucial as you are repairing these pathways.

JOURNAL

The trends in your serum blood sugar can tell you a lot about what you need to do for repair. Be a chronic tester; if you test your blood sugar, chart it, ideally, for three months. Look at what your blood sugar is before you eat, but also one and two hours after eating. Show these results to your doctor—this can be valuable information. It can also reveal what happens when you eat particular things, or don't eat, and how those factors affect your blood sugar. Remember, you are striving for stability, stability, stability! Blood sugar should spike after a meal, but should normalize in one to two hours and be lower in the morning than it is before bed. So, look at it before you go to bed and look at it first thing in the morning. It should not spike before a meal. If it is not acting normally, consider what you were eating or whether you ate at all. If you have received a diagnosis of prediabetes or diabetes, and you don't have a blood testing kit but you are interested in doing this, ask your doctor about its usefulness for you and how to get one through your insurance. Or, you can easily get blood glucose testing equipment online or at your local pharmacy. I use this method with many of my PCOS (polycystic ovarian syndrome) clients to check blood sugar values through different phases of their cycles. You and your doctor may have decided that this is not necessary, but it is a great tool and an additional way to listen to the body. There is a lot of work going into development of new equipment that won't require needle sticks, including one technology that beams light through the skin. Look for that soon!

BRIEFING YOUR DREAM TEAM

Doctors often run a fasting blood sugar test, but I also like to see a fasting insulin test, because if one of these is high, the other should be high as well. If the blood sugar is on the high end of normal and insulin is on the low end of normal, they might still both be "normal," but to me this would signal an impending problem with blood sugar.

If your doctor suspects diabetes, there are certain tests that you will most certainly undergo, because they are required for diagnosing it (the tests are slightly different for children, or to diagnose type 1 diabetes, and/or gestational diabetes mellitus in pregnant women):

- A1C

- Fasting plasma glucose test (FPG)

- Oral glucose tolerance test

Remember, you want to partner with your doctor. In any good relationship, the *why* is necessary, so be sure the doctor knows your symptoms and write down your test requests! The above tests may be all your doctor does to give you a definitive diagnosis of diabetes or prediabetes, but it's helpful to get some additional information. I recommend asking for these additional tests:

- **Fasting insulin:** Insulin helps transport glucose, the body's main source of energy. This test measures the amount of insulin in your blood after an eight- to twelve-hour fast.

- **Leptin:** Leptin is a hormone that maintains energy balance in the body by regulating metabolism and hunger. It helps your brain know when you are hungry or full. It's possible to lose sensitivity to leptin and have problems identifying hunger.

- **Adiponectin:** Adiponectin is a hormone released by fat cells that helps your body use both sugar and fat from food.

- **Aldosterone:** Aldosterone is a hormone released by the adrenal glands that helps the body regulate blood pressure. If your levels of this hormone are not within the normal range, it can lead to hard-to-control blood pressure or low blood pressure upon standing. Your levels also vary when standing, sitting, and lying down, or with salt intake, so ask your doctor about your test results. Sugar distribution is affected by both the liver and the muscle's ability to store glucose, and this hormone can give an indication of the efficiency or lack of efficiency of this pathway.

- **ACTH test:** Adrenocorticotropic hormone is a hormone released from the pituitary gland in the brain. It helps regulate blood pressure as well as blood sugar. This test can help pinpoint if your pituitary and adrenal glands are overproducing or underproducing. Levels change throughout the day, so it's recommended to have this test in the morning.

- **Urinalysis:** This can indicate issues with the kidneys or a diabetic condition. The test looks at the levels of ketones and protein in the urine.

SOMETHING TO CHEW ON

The important factor concerning diabetes and blood sugar issues is to embrace the idea that you have to eat because you are starving on a cellular level. Repairing the mechanism of delivery and acceptance of nutrients into the cell will shift that, but it is necessary to eat. Yet, don't label yourself as "starving." I tell a lot of my clients with prediabetes, insulin resistance, and PCOS to shift that "I'm starving" thought to "I'm waiting for food delivery." Take a few minutes, breathe deeply, calm yourself, and don't panic about being ravenous. Remind yourself that your food will be delivered through your cells, and then sit down and eat.

CHAPTER 11

Immune Dysfunction and Autoimmune Disorders

This is a special chapter for me, because I have an autoimmune disorder. It is also a chapter that is difficult to write. I know exactly what it's like to have a body that wages war on itself. When I was a student and I was first diagnosed with an autoimmune disease, that diagnosis changed the whole course of my life. I abandoned my lifelong dream of becoming a veterinarian. I had to do that because this diagnosis radically changed how I was living my life. Instead, I had to focus all my energy on learning about the biochemistry of the human body so I could figure out how to fix myself. I took classes and seminars, and I read obsessively—anything I thought would be relevant to what I needed to know. I drove my professors crazy asking questions and signing up for research projects. I was driven, I was on a mission to survive. I needed to understand: Why would my immune system turn on itself? Why couldn't I survive without being on prednisone? I studied the drug, its mechanism. I grew well versed in ANA titers and sedimentation rates, antiplatelet antibodies, and the host of nutrients, cofactors, coenzymes, and mechanisms that made the immune system work.

An autoimmune disease is a disease in which the body's immune system overreacts and begins attacking the body. It can attack any part, any organ; and the kind of autoimmune disease it is—the diagnosis—is largely related to what part of the body is (or what systems are) being attacked. There are many autoimmune conditions. Here are just a few:

- Addison's disease

- Celiac disease

- Graves' disease

- Hashimoto's thyroiditis

- Lupus

- Multiple sclerosis

- Psoriasis

- Rheumatoid arthritis

- Scleroderma

- Sjogren's syndrome

- Vitaligo

Additionally, there's nonspecific autoimmune disease—what they call it when they aren't sure what exact autoimmune process is happening.

Having an autoimmune disease is confusing, frustrating, and physically insulting. Autoimmunity almost seems symbolic: a body literally turning on itself and thereby lacking confidence in its own trustworthiness.

We all know of a few autoimmune diseases; rheumatoid arthritis and lupus are common ones. However, research continues to speculate and confirm that diseases we once thought were caused by other factors (or whose causes we didn't understand) are actually by-products of autoimmunity: type 1 diabetes, multiple sclerosis, celiac disease, psoriasis, inflammatory bowel syndrome. There are even some researchers who believe that heart disease, cancer, and dementia might have autoimmune components.[22, 23]

Science is desperately researching possible causes of specific autoimmune disorders. Can a pathogen, like a parasite, or a viral or bacterial infection trigger an autoimmune disorder? Or might a toxic substance such as chemicals, heavy metals, or pesticides be the cause? Often, there is an endless feedback loop: The body's immune system may turn itself on after getting overly excited by a virus or cancer, or an autoimmune condition could damage the heart and result in heart disease. Recent research suggests that autoimmune diseases like multiple sclerosis could be due to a metabolic disorder involving faulty fat metabolism rather than autoimmunity.

But if we are to believe that metabolic pathways regulate immunity, aren't they really one and the same? To me, these are not mutually exclusive; it's that feedback loop again. Which came first, the faulty metabolism or the autoimmunity? Which came first, the predisposition to an autoimmune disease or the susceptibility to a virus? Could the exposure to a virus trigger inflammation, which then disrupts the metabolism, which overexcites the immune system? Could a person's body have a genetic predisposition to compromised detoxification pathways, making that body the canary in the coal mine? All of these are possibilities and probabilities, but the reaction is the same: We have to "unset" the stage for these diseases and disrupt what was a perfect storm.

Science is still, and always will be, unraveling the complexities of human biochemistry. We have much to learn about autoimmunity and where it fits into the network of our body's actions and reactions. The bottom line—and the aspect that is so unsettling about autoimmunity, no matter the cause or the mechanism—is that the body's systems that are designed to work efficiently sometimes go awry and instead make us sick—chronically sick, and sometimes seemingly irreversibly sick, sending us in a downward spiral that seems impossible to escape. Autoimmunity is a perfect storm, created by the convergence of too many negative influences. The body, it seems, becomes confused, attempting to resolve the issue while mistakenly destroying itself in the process.

If you have a history of allergies, whether they are inhalant allergies or food allergies, that is a sign of a dysfunction in the immune system. If you are chronically stressed, that compromises your body's ability to adapt to immune stressors. If you get an infection, whether viral or something like Lyme disease, that can cause your immune system to come out swinging. All of these could become triggers. You can do something about all of this, however. You can adapt and manipulate your metabolism using the natural rhythm of the body in conjunction with targeted micronutrients to set your immune system back on track.

THE SELF-DISCOVERY ZONE

You might already know you have an autoimmune disorder, or maybe you just suspect it. Autoimmunity is hard to diagnose because it manifests itself in a thousand different ways, but there are some common threads. Suspect autoimmunity if this list of symptoms as a group seems familiar to you or if you have a lot of them:

- ANA titers and/or rheumatoid factors that are positive

- Balance and/or coordination issues

- Brain fog (one of the most common autoimmune symptoms)

- Chronic pain

- Concentration issues

- Diagnosis of an autoimmune disorder

- Dry eyes

- Dry mouth

- Eczema, psoriasis, or unexplained skin rashes

- Elevated sed rate and/or CRP levels

- Fatigue

- Fever

- Joint pain with swelling not related to injury, especially joint pain that is symmetrical (such as in both wrists or both ankles)

- Loss of self—the feeling that you aren't yourself, or that everything you knew about yourself has disappeared

- Mobility issues, like foot drag or unexplained clumsiness

- Numbness and tingling in any part of your body

- Swollen glands

DEALING, NOT HEALING

The conventional view of autoimmune disorders is that we aren't totally sure why they happen. Fair enough. But the way doctors have traditionally been taught to treat autoimmunity is to suppress, or sometimes even totally shut down, your body's immune system. This makes sense in a narrow sort of way. If the immune system is getting too excited, calming it down by muzzling it could stop the damage it is doing. It probably won't surprise you to learn that the protocol of choice to do this involves immunosuppressive medication.

The problem with this standard approach is that you need your immune system! This is why these drugs have so many warnings on them. If your over-active immune system is suddenly suppressed, it can't do the work to protect you from all the environmental pathogens out there, from the flu virus to a kidney infection. If you have an autoimmune disease, your doctor might also give you steroids, to bring down inflammation. Your adrenal gland should be secreting these, but may not be doing enough in the case of autoimmunity.

Depending on the autoimmune condition you have, you might also get some dietary prescriptions. For example, if you have celiac disease, your body attacks itself when exposed to gluten, the protein in wheat. People with celiac

---

WHAT SCIENCE SAYS IS TRUE

According to a report from the National Institutes of Health, "Most autoimmune diseases disproportionately affect women, and autoimmune diseases are among the 10 leading causes of death for women in every age group up to 64 years of age. All ages are affected, with onset from childhood to late adulthood," and autoimmune disease prevalence—including lupus, multiple sclerosis, celiac disease, and type 1 diabetes—is increasing.* There are many theories about why this is happening, including changes in diet, modification of our food supply, increased stress levels, changes in the gut's microbial environment, exposure to environmental toxins, and genetic influences. I believe these are all probably influencing the growing incidence of autoimmunity.

---

* National Institutes of Health Autoimmune Diseases Coordinating Committee, Progress in Autoimmune Diseases Research Report to Congress, U.S. Department of Health and Human Services, March 2005, https://www.niaid.nih.gov/topics/autoimmune/Documents/adccfinal.pdf.

disease absolutely cannot eat gluten for the rest of their lives without risk of severe symptoms and internal damage, including a much higher chance of developing cancer of the small intestine. There is some evidence that a gluten-free diet can ease symptoms in some other autoimmune diseases, too.

Yet, while there is much talk about pharmaceutical approaches, there is very little talk about how diet might help to regulate and boost the mechanisms that correct and balance immunity in the human body. I'm not talking about eliminating a particular food or food component when it is a problem for a particular autoimmune condition. I am talking about a global dietary approach to immunity. I'm talking about stopping the autoimmune boulder from rolling down the hill. I've done it in my own body, so I know it can be done.

TARGETED PATHWAYS FOR REPAIR

Because of my own experience, I am obsessed with taking a step back and asking: "Why is this happening?" What would make a perfectly sound body suddenly attack itself? What would send the immune system into overdrive? And how can we reverse that process?

When people have autoimmune disorders, their bodies are overwhelmed. It's like someone's jumping into bed in the middle of the day and pulling the covers over her head and saying, "I just can't deal with it. I can't cope. I have a list of ten things to do and I don't know where to start!" Your body adapts to the environment in which you place it, but each body has its boiling point. Our environments are already full of viruses, bacteria, and carcinogens, not to mention events that stress both our bodies and our minds, from sleep deprivation to work stress to family drama.

Normally, we can handle the constant onslaught, and our immune systems dispatch the troublemakers fairly easily. When we overload our body's capacity to manage its issues, however, the body can get worn down, the adrenals can get exhausted, the immune system can panic—and then it all goes haywire. When that one virus, one tragic event, or one toxic exposure becomes one too many, it can be the straw that breaks the camel's back; that's all it takes to tip us into a full-blown attack on the self.

It's no wonder we jump (metaphorically) into that warm, safe bed and pull the covers up over our heads. But rather than dragging you out of bed, or trying to talk you out of your attitude, or telling you to just snap out of it, I want to crack the door open, peek inside, and whisper, "Hey, if I handle seven of the things on your list, do you think you could handle the other three?"

With autoimmunity, it's really about listening to your body and figuring out what is causing that stress, then striking a balance. This lowers the body's overstimulated reactivity response. The things I target with an autoimmune prescription are:

- Glucocorticoids (stress hormones) that regulate immunity, delving deeper into that particular steroid hormone

- The metabolic pathways that regulate prostaglandins, the pro- and anti-inflammatory hormones

- The metabolic pathways that regulate "allergic" responses in the body (part of the immune modulation)

- The pathways that create a homeostasis in the spleen, bone marrow, and mineral distribution, which are sending mixed messages to the immune system

To address these, first, we eliminate the most common things likely to be reactors. For example, with autoimmune clients, I always have an eye out for food allergies, signs of heavy-metal toxicity, and gluten reactions because these are common to autoimmunity. I also look for latent viral infections, like Epstein-Barr virus and Lyme disease, which also are often linked to autoimmune reactivity. Something is impacting the immune system, therefore reducing some common triggers can often start to calm things down so we can get to the heart of what's really going on.

Next, I look at where the attack is focused. What part of the body is getting victimized? Is it the blood? The joints? The skin? The GI tract? The nervous system? This answer can help in designing a food prescription. Finally, is there a genetic predisposition to an autoimmune condition? Having one autoimmune disorder can make you more likely to have another, and a family history of an autoimmune disorder could be a sign that you are genetically predisposed to another condition, not necessarily to the one your mother or brother or aunt or cousin has.

Finally, I make a peace plan. If the body is attacking itself, it's time to intervene and stop the war.

REMOVE, REPAIR, AND RESTORE

I had lofty goals for myself when I was diagnosed at age nineteen, and I have lofty goals for you, too:

1. Remove obstacles in the pathways for detoxification, including viruses. This is like opening the windows and doors in the spring to let out all the stale winter air. People with autoimmunity tend to have a high toxin load, and it is important to get these toxins out of the system so the body can work properly again. We will also remove, or at least address, mild latent infections and toxicity loads that have disrupted metabolic pathways that regulate hormones, as well as disrupted the neurotransmitters that affect the skin and sensory organs, creating multisensory reactions in the body.

2. Repair the body's focused mission of attack and the blood sugar modulation issues and carbohydrate resistance that are worsening the situation.

3. Restore calm to the body by nourishing the adrenals and correcting the imbalance in the adrenal fight-or-flight hormones, which disrupt the body's natural steroid and anti-inflammation hormones. Ideally, we get to the heart of what is upsetting the body by looking at the symptoms; but even if we never find out for sure, just calming the body, psychologically and physiologically, can help the immune system settle down. That means a targeted effort to remove stressors, from an overextended schedule to foods that stress digestion.

GUIDELINES FOR YOUR IMMUNE REPAIR RX

To get the most from your Immune Repair prescription, follow these principles:

- You will be taking this prescription six times a day (eating six times a day). That means you will have three strategic immune-balancing meals every day, plus three targeted immune-balancing snacks every day. Notice that with this meal plan, you don't start with breakfast. Your snack comes first in the morning. You will take your prescription (eat) every three to four hours while you are awake.

- This prescription introduces the concept of food rotation. This isn't something I've talked about in any of my other books, and it may be a new concept for you, but basically you will not eat any one food more than three times per week, and preferably never two days in a row. The meal map will help you achieve this. Notice that unlike any other week, this week switches plans back and forth to help you maintain a rotation diet. You will eat in one style for days 1 and 5 (Monday and Friday). You will eat in a different way on days 2 through 4 and 6 and 7 (the rest of the week).

- Many people begin to notice results in their symptom profile within thirty days, but for me, this eating style is one that I employ any time I know I will be under extreme stress. I've had extra exposures, I've been sick, anything that could trigger the propensity to create a flare-up in my immune system. But for the first time you do this, stay on it for eight to twelve months.

- If you object to any of the foods on this plan for any reason, just replace them with a different food from the Foundational Foods List and the Top 20 Power Foods for Immune Repair list. For example, you could substitute apricots for blueberries or cucumber for jícama. However, be sure to notice that there is an Avoid list for this program as well. Even if a food is on the Foundational Foods List, do not eat it if it also appears on the Avoid list for this particular prescription.

- Tell your doctor that you are working on dietary strategies to help stabilize your immune system, and ask for the lab tests I recommend at the end of this chapter, so you can have a more specific idea of where you stand and so you can monitor your progress on this prescription. This approach could necessitate alterations in your medications, so always keep your doctor in the loop.

- Carry your food list and meal map with you wherever you go so you are always able to have an immune-balancing meal or snack at the right time.

Autoimmunity can be influenced by genetics, infection, toxicity, emotions, or all of these. Environmental changes create an ecosystem that's ripe for autoimmunity, and the diversity of the dysfunction requires diversity in treatment. Therefore, the food prescription also requires a certain diversity, and the best way I have found to tackle this problem is with a rotation diet.

Rotation diets are good for managing food allergies and for nutrient diversity, but they are absolutely essential for people with autoimmune disease. A rotation diet works on the principle that even the healthiest foods can become dysfunctional if they are eaten too often, so all foods are staggered; no one food is repeated more than three times a week.

Here are the principles:

- Look at the meal map and the Top 20 Power Foods list, and also look at the Avoid list in this chapter. Make a list of all the foods you plan to or are likely to eat that week. Keep it on the refrigerator. Every time you eat something, make a check mark or an X next to that item. When you have three checks or Xs, you are done eating that food until next week. Choose something else from the list.
- The meal map is set up to help you. For example, you will have complex carbs with vegetables on certain days and proteins with vegetables on certain days.
- Never eat complex carbs and proteins together. In people with autoimmune issues, the combination of carbs and protein can create a firestorm of acidosis and trigger the hormones of inflammation.
- Always eat fruit on an empty stomach, and wait thirty minutes before eating anything else.
- Grocery shop strategically. For example, during the first week, you will need fourteen pieces of fruit, but no more than three servings of any one fruit. You can put your servings in your own separate fruit bowl to select from during the week.
- If you have to purchase a larger size (such as a bag of apples), put your fruit in a separate location. I make my bowl of fruit for the week and

> leave the rest in the refrigerator for my family. You can also freeze extra
> portions of food for upcoming weeks.
> - Because complex carbs are only recommended two times a week, on
>   days 1 and 5 you will need a total of four servings of complex carbs. I
>   recommend my clients choose a minimum of two different kinds each
>   week. For example, you might have two servings of gluten-free oat-
>   meal and two servings of sprouted adzuki beans (order these online—
>   they are worth it and so good for your immune system!).
> - Pay attention to the Avoid list!

EAT YOUR MEDICINE: YOUR IMMUNE REPAIR RX

Are you ready to be your body's peacemaker? In addition to the rotation diet, the nutritional prescription for autoimmunity must remove reactors that trigger the immune system to overreact, repair stress, and restore calm.

If you have an autoimmune disease, it is important to eliminate the most common triggers from your diet. Pay close attention to the Avoid list. Even though these items are on the Foundational Foods List, they are not good for *you*. You might not react to them all, but many people with autoimmunity have become so reactive and sensitive that they have inflammatory responses to foods they might otherwise do fine with once their systems have calmed down.

Also, be careful with, and go easy on, all grain-based carbohydrates, even if they don't contain gluten. That includes rice, oats, and quinoa.

Notice that, in the morning, you will be having fruit within thirty minutes of waking, and no other food for thirty more minutes. At night, you will be having fruit within thirty minutes of bedtime, and then no other food until morning. This is important because fruit contains fructose, so it can ferment in the gut and excite the immune system. When eaten alone, the body seems to be able to digest it more efficiently, not alerting the immune system to react. That's why we start and end the day with fruit, with the hope that the stomach is the most empty at those two times of day. However, don't avoid fruit entirely. Although fruits need to be eaten alone, the natural sugars are nurturing to the adrenal glands, which help regulate immune function.

TOP 20 POWER FOODS FOR IMMUNE REPAIR

Apricots	Cucumbers
Arugula	Garlic
Asparagus	Jícama
Beef liver (organic)	Olives
Blueberries	Radishes
Brussels sprouts	Sardines
Butternut squash	Sprouted adzuki beans
Cauliflower	Sweet potatoes
Celery	Turkey
Cranberries	Watermelon

The first thing to review is your Top 20 Power Foods list and the Avoid list that are so important for your diet. Use these power foods to feed your body and encourage repair of an overactive immune system. Favor these foods and then fill in the rest of your meal map with foods from the Foundational Foods List, except for the Avoid foods.

My strategy for the first and fifth days of this plan is to introduce complex carbs into the body to support carbohydrate metabolism and create a diversity in micronutrients. They need to be introduced in a way that is as non-insulting as possible. Carbs are typically acidifying, which can make them inflammatory triggers, so you will never eat them with flesh-based protein, which can also be acidifying. However, carbs eaten with vegetables alkalize the body; you more readily break down the carbohydrates without stimulating the immune component of inflammation. But even so, this is difficult for a body dealing with an autoimmune disorder, which is why you do it twice a week, and only when separated by days that include no grain-based carbohydrates.

Remember—no complex carbs with protein, and only eat fruit on an empty stomach!

Although the foods on this list are generally considered nutritious, they can be triggers for autoimmunity. If this is your challenge, temporarily cross these foods off your Foundational Foods List:

Almonds

Cherries

Chiles and peppers, including all sweet and hot chiles and peppers like bell, banana, frying peppers, jalapeños, pimientos, and habanero; as well as spices made from peppers, like paprika and cayenne (black pepper is okay)

Eggplant

Eggs

Goji berries

White potatoes (sweet potatoes are okay)

Rice

Sprouted grain, spelt, and Kamut (only if you have celiac disease or gluten intolerance)

Tomatillos

Tomatoes

Anyone with an autoimmune disorder must carefully read ingredients and look for hidden gluten, dairy, corn, rice, potatoes, and soy products. These are common triggers for autoimmunity, and although you won't be intentionally eating them because they aren't on your Foundational Foods List, they are commonly hidden in prepared foods. Products labeled "gluten-free" are not necessarily safe, as they often contain dairy, corn, rice, potatoes, or soy.

MEAL MAP FOR IMMUNE REPAIR, DAYS 1 AND 5

SNACK	BREAKFAST	LUNCH	SNACK	DINNER	SNACK
Fruit (high or low G.I.) within ½ hour of waking; nothing else for ½ hour	Complex Carb Vegetable (green)	Protein Vegetable Healthy Fat	Complex Carb Vegetable (green)	Protein Vegetable Healthy Fat	Fruit (high or low G.I.) within ½ hour of bedtime; no other food!

My strategy for days 2 to 4 and days 6 and 7—the remaining days—is to pull out all the complex carbs. On these days, protein is the focus. Protein is important for adrenal stabilization and regulating the glucocorticoid pathways, which control steroid production. Remember, synthetic steroids are often the therapy of choice for autoimmune disorders. Balancing these steroids naturally in the body can be powerful medicine as well.

MEAL MAP FOR IMMUNE REPAIR, DAYS 2–4 AND 6–7

SNACK	BREAKFAST	LUNCH	SNACK	DINNER	SNACK
Fruit (high or low G.I.) within ½ hour of waking; nothing else for ½ hour	Protein Vegetable	Protein Vegetable Healthy Fat	Fruit (high or low G.I.) Vegetable	Protein Vegetable Healthy Fat	Fruit (high or low G.I.) within ½ hour of bedtime; no other food!

A DAY IN THE LIFE OF IMMUNE REPAIR

Here is an example of how you might use the food lists to create your own meal plan following the meal map for Immune Repair prescription. The first is an example of how you might choose to eat during days 1 or 5, and the second is an example of how you might choose to eat during days 2 through 4 or 6 and 7. Recipes that follow appear in boldface in the meal map.

SAMPLE DAY MAP FOR IMMUNE REPAIR, DAYS 1 AND 5

SNACK	BREAKFAST	LUNCH	SNACK	DINNER	SNACK
Blueberries	**Veggie Bagel** (see Note)	**Smoked Salmon Salad**	Sprouted adzuki beans wrapped in butter lettuce leaves	**Filet Mignon with Green Beans**	Apricots

RECIPES

VEGGIE BAGEL

Serves 2

    8 fresh basil leaves
    2 teaspoons cider vinegar
    1 teaspoon nutritional yeast
    Sea salt
    Freshly ground black pepper
    1 sprouted-grain bagel, cut in half
    ½ cup thinly sliced cucumber
    1 cup trimmed fresh spinach

NOTE: If you have celiac disease or are gluten-free, replace the sprouted-grain bagel with a gluten-free tortilla, or put these veggies over ½ cup of quinoa.

Either in a food processor or using a knife, chop and blend the basil leaves, vinegar, and nutritional yeast until smooth, then season to taste with salt and pepper.

Toast the bagel halves and spread both with the basil spread. Top with cucumber slices and spinach leaves.

SMOKED SALMON SALAD

Serves 2

    ½ tablespoon lemon juice
    ½ tablespoon coconut vinegar
    Sea salt
    Freshly ground black pepper
    2 tablespoons olive oil
    12 ounces smoked salmon, flaked
    2 cucumbers, cubed
    1 cup grated carrots
    1 cup grated zucchini
    6 cups romaine lettuce, torn or cut into bite-size pieces
    1 tablespoon chopped fresh parsley
    1 tablespoon chopped fresh thyme
    2 tablespoons chopped pecans

In a mixing bowl, whisk together the lemon juice, vinegar, and salt and pepper to taste. Slowly drizzle in the olive oil while whisking to form a vinaigrette.

In another bowl, toss together the salmon, cucumbers, carrots, zucchini, and lettuce. Add the herbs and pecans, then drizzle the dressing over and toss to coat well.

FILET MIGNON WITH GREEN BEANS

Serves 2

> 1 8-ounce filet mignon
> Sea salt
> Black pepper
> 4 tablespoons olive oil
> 2 cups trimmed and sliced green beans (1-inch pieces)
> 1 cup trimmed and quartered radishes
> 1 small shallot, thinly sliced
> 3 garlic cloves, thinly sliced
> 1 lemon, cut in half

Season the steak with salt and pepper to taste. Add 2 tablespoons of the olive oil to a heavy-bottomed skillet or cast-iron frying pan set over high heat. Add the filet and cook until the internal temperature reaches 130°F for rare, 135°F for medium, 145°F for medium well, and 155°F for well done. Remove from the pan and let rest for 5 minutes.

Using the same pan set over medium high heat, add the remaining 2 tablespoons olive oil, then the beans, radishes, shallot, garlic, and juice of half a lemon. Cook for 5 minutes or until vegetables are tender.

Serve the vegetable garnish alongside the steak and squeeze the remaining lemon half over it, if desired.

Now, here is a sample of how you could eat on days 2, 3, 4, 6, and 7. Recipes that follow are shown in boldface in the meal map.

SAMPLE MEAL MAP FOR DAYS 2–4 AND 6–7

SNACK	BREAKFAST	LUNCH	SNACK	DINNER	SNACK
Watermelon cubes	**Cucumber Submarine Sandwich**	**Brussels Sprout Salad**	Blueberries and raw cauliflower florets	**Pork Chop with Cauliflower**	Smoothie made with cranberries, ice, and stevia or xylitol to sweeten

MORNING AND EVENING SNACKS

During days 1 and 5 (and also for the rest of the week), your morning and evening snacks will consist of fruit only. In the morning, remember to have fruit within thirty minutes of waking, and no other food for thirty more minutes. At night, remember to have fruit within thirty minutes of bedtime, and then no other food until morning. This is very important! Please do not deviate from this crucial part of your prescription.

- Watermelon
- Raspberries
- Peaches
- Any combination of allowed fruits blended with water and ice into a smoothie

AFTERNOON SNACK

As the meal map states, this snack should contain a complex carb and a green vegetable on days 1 and 5.

- Gluten-free sprouted-grain toast with butter lettuce leaves
- White beans mashed and packed into celery sticks
- Gluten-free crackers with cucumber slices

RECIPES

CUCUMBER SUBMARINE SANDWICH

Serves 1

¼ cup alfalfa sprouts

¼ cup trimmed arugula

1 tablespoon lemon juice

Sea salt

Freshly ground black pepper

4 ounces deli-sliced turkey breast

1 English cucumber, trimmed and cut in half lengthwise, any seeds removed

Combine the alfalfa sprouts and arugula in a bowl. Sprinkle with the lemon juice and season to taste with salt and pepper. Toss well.

Lay the turkey slices on one half of the cucumber. Top with the arugula mixture. Place the other cucumber half on top and close the sandwich.

BRUSSELS SPROUT SALAD

Serves 2

4 tablespoons olive oil, divided
8 ounces boneless, skinless chicken breast
Sea salt
Black pepper
1 pound Brussels sprouts, cored and leaves separated
$1/2$ cup grated carrot
$1/4$ cup thinly sliced celery (about $1/2$ rib)
1 tablespoon champagne vinegar or white wine vinegar
2 teaspoons whole-grain mustard
2 teaspoons stevia
1 teaspoon lemon juice
$1/4$ teaspoon grated lemon zest
1 tablespoon chopped pecans

Prepare a grill or preheat a grill pan.

Brush 1 tablespoon of the oil on the chicken and then season it with $1/2$ teaspoon each salt and pepper. Place on the grill and grill for 5 to 6 minutes, turning once, until cooked through and the internal temperature reaches 165°F. Let the chicken rest for 5 minutes, then cut into $1/2$-inch cubes.

In a large salad bowl, combine the chicken, the Brussels sprout leaves, carrot, and celery.

In a small bowl, whisk together the olive oil, vinegar, mustard, stevia, lemon juice, and zest. Season the dressing to taste with salt and pepper. Drizzle the dressing over the salad and toss to coat. Refrigerate for 30 minutes.

Garnish the salad with chopped pecans.

PORK CHOP WITH CAULIFLOWER

Serves 2

    Sea salt
    Freshly ground black pepper
    1 cauliflower, cored and cut into florets
    4 tablespoons olive oil
    1 tablespoon lemon juice
    3 garlic cloves, minced
    1 tablespoon ground cumin
    1 tablespoon ground coriander
    1 teaspoon chopped fresh thyme
    1/2 teaspoon chopped fresh oregano
    1 8-ounce boneless pork chop
    2 teaspoons sliced fresh chives

Preheat the oven to 450°F.

In a bowl, toss the cauliflower with 1½ tablespoons of the olive oil, the lemon juice, and ½ teaspoon each salt and pepper. Toss well, then spread the cauliflower on a baking sheet and roast for 20 to 25 minutes, or until lightly browned. Use a fork to test for doneness; the tines should easily pierce the cauliflower when done.

Mix the garlic, cumin, coriander, thyme, oregano, and 1½ tablespoons olive oil in a small bowl, then season with salt and pepper. Rub the paste onto the pork chop.

Heat the remaining tablespoon of oil in a medium sauté pan over high heat and sauté the chop about 5 minutes on each side, or until the internal temperature reaches 145°F.

Slice the chop in half and place on plates. Garnish with the chives.

MORNING AND EVENING SNACKS

For all days of the week, your morning snack will consist of fruit only. In the morning, remember to have fruit within thirty minutes of waking and no other food for thirty more minutes. At night, remember to have fruit within thirty minutes of bedtime and then no other food until morning.

- Apple
- Blackberries
- Oranges
- Cranberry smoothie blended with lime juice and stevia

AFTERNOON SNACK

As the meal map states, this snack should contain a fruit and a vegetable on days 2 through 4 and 6 and 7.

- Oranges and jícama sticks
- Peaches and carrot sticks
- Kiwi slices and celery

RESTORE IMMUNE SYSTEM BALANCE: TOP THREE NON-FOOD STRATEGIES

Food is the linchpin of immune repair, but there are many other things you can do to support your nutritional prescription. These are some of my favorites.

REDUCE STRESS

One of the most important things you can do for yourself if you have an immune disease is to reduce your stress. Autoimmunity is about overreaction, so don't mirror that in your life. For me, that means riding my horse. It helps me so much that I think my health insurance should cover it! When I do it regularly, I know (because I journal and get my labs done so often) that there is a direct correlation between riding time and lower ANA titers. For you, it can be anything that takes stress off your plate. If that's singing, join a choir. If that's yoga, you can't let anything trivial take precedence over getting to that class. If it's painting, join or start one of those painting groups, or take lessons, or just make time to do it *often*. These are lifesaving measures. Stress hormones are a catalyst for an overactive immune system. If it brings you joy and removes your stress, *do it*. It has to be part of your life.

PTSD THERAPY

Having an autoimmune disease is traumatic. It can feel as if someone has broken into your intimate home—the home of your soul—and stolen something. You can feel violated, betrayed, as if the place you thought was the safest in the world is not safe at all. Repatterning therapies work well for people who have autoimmune disease, especially those used to treat post-traumatic stress disorder (PTSD). One of my favorites is EMDR. EMDR stands for Eye Movement Desensitization and Reprocessing, and it is a type of psychotherapy that involves eight phases of information processing. It is simple to learn and involves image recall, and following with your eyes certain motions the therapist makes. If you aren't familiar with it, it probably sounds kind of weird, but it is highly effective. Other types of therapies that are great for both PTSD and people with autoimmune disease are neurofeedback, cognitive behavioral therapy, and support groups. A support group can be a double-edged sword, however, if hearing about the extreme experiences of others makes you feel worse. But if you like the idea of being with people having the same struggles, this could be a great release. It's nice to experience common understanding, but just remember that nobody else's story is your story. You author your autobiography.

IV NUTRITIONALS

I am a huge advocate of IV nutritionals like methylated B vitamins and glutathione to support my liver and help to create homeostasis in my immune function. This treatment involves going to the doctor and getting an IV that infuses you with the supportive substances. I credit some of my personal success to use of preservative-free IV nutritionals. I started these therapies when I was twenty-one years old and I still use them. They were difficult to find back then, but are much more common now. Be aware, though, that many conventional doctors don't use them, and those who do often use infusions that are full of preservatives and corn by-products. If you want to try this treatment, find a physician who is either in the American College for Advancement in Medicine (ACAM) or the Institute of Functional Medicine (IFM), or who is a naturopathic doctor and can verify that the infusions are preservative and additive free.

BRIEFING YOUR DREAM TEAM

If your doctor suspects you have an autoimmune disease, you will probably be given certain standard tests, which look for the markers of an overly active immune system. Make sure you keep a list of any active symptoms, and put those in writing every time you visit your physician, especially when you request lab tests. You want to give your doctor all the ammunition he or she needs to order the tests you want. These are the tests I recommend. Your doctor may already plan to order some of these, but see how many more you can get:

PRIMARY TESTS:
These are the most important tests to get.

- **ANA (antinuclear antibody):** This test detects antibodies to certain antigens. It can suggest an autoimmune disease, although it isn't very specific about which one. A normal test result will reveal no ANA in the blood. It's not exactly a diagnostic test, but it is evidence that points toward autoimmunity.

- **ESR (erythrocyte sedimentation rate):** This test is another measure of inflammation.

- **Rheumatoid factor (RF):** This is a specific test for rheumatoid arthritis but may also be present with lupus, Sjogren's syndrome, and several other autoimmune conditions.

- **Aldolase:** This is a really great marker, especially in those who have tissue modulation like scleroderma or other skin issues. Aldolase is an enzyme that breaks down sugars to produce energy. It is found in high amounts in muscle tissue.

- **C-reactive protein (CRP):** This test measures inflammation and can identify flare-ups of inflammatory diseases like rheumatoid arthritis or lupus.

- **Immunoglobulin:** This test indicates serum Ig levels, especially IgG, IgA, and IgM, which can show how well the immune system is working.

SECONDARY TESTS:

Your doctor may be less familiar with or willing to run these tests, but a functional medicine or naturopathic doctor may be more open to doing so. Ask your doctor if these are available to you:

- **Anti-cyclic citrullinated peptide antibody:** This is a test for a biomarker for rheumatoid arthritis but may also be present in cases of juvenile arthritis, psoriatic arthritis, lupus, Sjogren's syndrome, and other autoimmune conditions. Like the ANA test, this is a marker used along with other markers to make a diagnosis of autoimmunity.

- **Anti-double stranded DNA (anti-dsDNA):** This tests for antibodies that, when present, may indicate lupus in particular.

- **Enzyme-linked immunosorbent assay (ELISA):** This detects and measures specific antibodies that could indicate an upset immune system.

- **Lyme, Epstein-Barr, and cytomegalovirus:** These tests show the presence of their respective conditions.

The following two tests are wonderful to know about because they are so easy to support if your result is positive, and they can be life-changing when nutritionally supported. If you can do these tests easily, do them. If there is an abnormal value, all you have to do is take methylated folic acid or a transdermal or IV glutathione supplement. Both these tests can be done with a simple cheek swab.

- **MTHFR:** This test determines whether you have a genetic mutation that makes it difficult for you to metabolize folate and can indicate many complicated health issues.

- **Glutathione insufficiency:** This test determines whether you have a disorder that prevents your body from producing glutathione. This can cause cell damage, anemia, and in severe cases, seizures and other neurological symptoms.

SOMETHING TO CHEW ON

A lot of people with autoimmune disorders come to my clinic. Curiously, when I was writing my first book and I made the decision to move from the clinic to a larger community, I had to trust that it would be successful—but it was very difficult for me to trust myself. Similarly, this is a challenge for people with autoimmunity. We lose trust in our body's ability to make the right decisions healthwise, and it therefore becomes difficult to trust our own judgment.

For instance, when things creep up, even something like a common cold, it's easy to freak out, thinking all your progress has disappeared and you are back where you started. *Oh, my God, I'm having another flare!* When you have an autoimmune disease, you know exactly what your body has the capacity to do and where it could take you, and you don't want to go there. But it is even more damaging to let that fear overcome you.

Don't be afraid to dance again, to love again, to trust again. Don't be afraid to view your body as healthy and vibrant and alive. Don't be afraid to trust your body—because even if you never know everything about the why, you know your body did and it will continue to do whatever is the best job it knows how to do in order to take care of you at any given moment.

I gain so much inspiration watching my clients get back out on the dance floor of life, even after extreme personal struggles, and it makes me want to get out there, too. They were willing to share their suffering, as well as their triumphs. Maybe you can find a way to do that, too—because it's a great way to live.

CHAPTER 12

Eat to Thrive

Miracles happen every day. Change your perception of what a miracle is,
and you'll see them all around you.

—Jon Bon Jovi

This has been an emotional book for me to write. I felt such intimacy with you, my reader, as I thought of so many people in my life who are struggling with these imbalances. Whether it is my niece, my sister, my dad, my brother-in-law, or my very best friend, I watch how feeding their bodies has nurtured their very quality of life. I also know firsthand how knocked down someone can feel when his or her body is out of balance or has manifested disease.

Maybe you want to start to restore balance, but you feel discouraged or completely devoid of hope. I get it. I've been there. In writing this book, I learned a lot about myself. I am always trying to repair the *why* in my body, and I tried to anticipate what you will need to be successful as well. But remember, this is a journey. I'm asking you to become enchanted with yourself. Be full of wonder and curiosity. That paradigm shift came at an early age for me. Maybe it was a coping mechanism, so I didn't give up on myself. Maybe by cooking and falling in love with food, I learned how to put the *fun* in *dysfunction*. Who really knows? What I do know is that I have witnessed real, clinical, meaningful change in my body and in the bodies of those I love deeply, as well as in the thousands of clients and hundreds of thousands of community members I call my tribe. And all of this has been done through the strategic use of food as medicine.

Don't forget that health is also harmony and happiness. I want you to be not just free of disease from a blood chemistry perspective but also free from the disease or the havoc that dysfunction can wreak in your life. I want you to feel in harmony. I want you to feel happy.

PICK YOUR STARTING POINT

Now that you have explored all seven food prescriptions, it's time to decide where you want to begin. Maybe you already know, or maybe you still aren't quite sure, because you have so many symptoms from so many different chapters. Don't be overwhelmed with the amount of information I've laid out. Put your toe in the water, and begin with the Self-Discovery Zones. Look at the Power Foods lists and start making some of the recipes that sound good to you.

At this point, I also encourage you to look back at the Health Wish List you made in Chapter 1. Keep that Health Wish List current. Cross off the old, but always look ahead. What are your new goals, your next goals, your *advanced health goals?* It's exciting to aim high, and to keep moving forward.

If you want even more definitive help, dig in and see where your body is telling you to start. In my clinic, the following is the exercise we use to help us determine where to potentially begin or where to go next. It is a living, breathing process that evolves as you explore the whys, so whenever you finish a prescription, try this test again to see where it leads to next. For now, for each question, check whether you almost always have this issue, whether you have it sometimes, or whether you almost never experience it.

And no matter what your results, remember that you are unique and special—and what a smart, smart body you have! It is quite possibly whispering in your ear, or telling you something, or even screaming from the rooftops. It is saying that it needs help, that it needs food. So let's listen together, and then step forward and answer.

YOUR WHOLE-BODY DIAGNOSIS QUIZ

Not quite sure where to start? Is your body sending you many messages, or some mixed messages? Fill out this questionnaire to determine where to begin. Then, each time you complete a prescription, if you want to dive back in, answer the questionnaire again to determine what to try next. You can also find a much more complete, definitive, and comprehensive digital quiz on my website, at www.hayliepomroy.com, if you want to go deeper. Score yourself based on this scale:

1 point—Never   2 points—Sometimes
3 points—Often   4 points—All the Time

QUESTIONS:

1. Do you have acid reflux or heartburn after eating or after going too long without eating?   1 2 3 4

2. Does your regular workout or the physical things you need to do each day suddenly feel harder or impossible? Does it even seem difficult to walk around the block?   1 2 3 4

3. Have you lost your sex drive, and/or for men, are you not having a morning erection?   1 2 3 4

4. Do you rarely sweat during exercise?   1 2 3 4

5. Do you have a ravenous appetite in the evening, after 5:00 p.m., or extreme sugar cravings in the afternoon?   1 2 3 4

6. Do you have an appetite that seems insatiable most of the time or excessive carbohydrate cravings?   1 2 3 4

7. Are you having sudden balance, coordination, or mobility issues?   1 2 3 4

8. Do you have bloating after eating, even to the extent of looking pregnant?   1 2 3 4

9. Are you falling asleep during the day, even at your desk, and/or having trouble getting to or staying asleep at night?   1 2 3 4

10. For women, has your menstrual cycle become heavier or clotty, and/or are your breasts tender or painful or changing in shape or density?   1 2 3 4

11. Is your appetite suddenly out of control?   1 2 3 4

12. Are you self-medicating with alcohol, food, or drugs to feel calm or interested in life?   1 2 3 4

13. Has your arm hair recently thickened or (for women) are you sprouting hairs on your chin, and/or are you losing the hair on your legs or toes or the crown of your head?   1 2 3 4

14. Do you have eczema, psoriasis, or unexplained rashes?   1 2 3 4

15. Do you have bowel movements that come out in long, thin ropes?   1 2 3 4

16. Do you experience pain that moves around your body, like a sensation of traveling bees?   1 2 3 4

17. Have you experienced rapid and sudden weight gain?   1 2 3 4

18. Do you have fat accumulation around your belly, abdomen, and/or waist (for example: a pot belly, beer belly, spare tire, or muffin top), or are you suddenly unable to zip up your jeans?   1 2 3 4

19. Do you have compulsive behaviors like knuckle cracking, hair twisting, or nail biting (or in more extreme cases, destructive behaviors like cutting or branding)?   1 2 3 4

20. Has your doctor told you that you have abnormal fasting blood sugar and/or insulin levels?   1 2 3 4

21. Do you have joint pain with swelling not related to an injury, especially symmetrical joint pain (such as in both wrists, hands, or ankles)?   1 2 3 4

22. Do you have frequent constipation or diarrhea (or do you alternate between the two?), and/or gas and flatulence?   1 2 3 4

23. Do you have daily sugar and/or carbohydrate cravings?   1 2 3 4

24. Are you experiencing mood swings, brain fog, and/or forgetfulness?   1 2 3 4

25. Has your doctor told you that your total cholesterol, LDL serum cholesterol, or triglycerides are too high, and/or that your HDL serum cholesterol is too low?   1 2 3 4

26. Are you having attention problems, hyperactivity issues, or a diagnosis of ADD or ADHD?   1 2 3 4

27. Are you experiencing tingling or numbness in your hands or feet?   1 2 3 4

28. Do you feel like you aren't yourself lately?   1 2 3 4

29. Do you have undigested food in your stool?   1 2 3 4

30. Do you feel like you are dragging through the day, or have fatigue all day long? Or do you have a profound energy slump in the middle of the afternoon?   1 2 3 4

31. Are you having hot flashes and/or night sweats?   1 2 3 4

32. Do you have creases in your earlobes?   1 2 3 4

33. Do you feel anxious or depressed, or have mood swings ranging from sadness or a loss of emotion to mania or other excessive emotions?   1 2 3 4

34. Has your doctor told you that you have positive ANA titers or rheumatoid factor?   1 2 3 4

35. Are you unusually thirsty and/or urinating more often than usual?   1 2 3 4

SCORING

Add your numbers for each group of questions below, and write down the totals.

Add questions 2, 9, 16, 23, and 30. This is your Energy score. _____

Add questions 4, 11, 18, 25, and 32. This is your Lipid score. _____

Add questions 6, 13, 20, 27, and 35. This is your Blood Sugar score. _____

Add questions 5, 12, 19, 26, and 33. This is your Mood/Cognition score. _____

Add questions 1, 8, 15, 22, and 29. This is your Gastrointestinal score. _____

Add questions 7, 14, 21, 28, and 34. This is your Autoimmunity score. _____

Add questions 3, 10, 17, 24, and 31. This is your Hormone score. _____

ANSWER KEY

Your score will range between 5 to 20 for each section. Use the point system below to determine which chapter's program is the highest priority for you now.

17–20 POINTS = High Priority Prescription: This is the area your body is telling you that you probably need to repair first. If you are having trouble deciding where to start, start here, as this symptom cluster is most prevalent and urgent. If you have more than one area that registers as High Priority, begin with the one that is the most uncomfortable or life-affecting, or that worries you the most—or the one that your doctor believes is most drastically impacting your health.

13–16 POINTS = Moderate Priority Prescription: This may be the issue to focus on next, or start here if these are the symptoms that bother you the most. Even though your score doesn't register as High Priority, you are still having issues in this area and can benefit from the nutritional plan.

9–12 POINTS = Low Priority Prescription: Although this registered as a low priority for you, you are still experiencing symptoms here and can benefit from following this chapter's nutritional plan, especially if these symptoms bother you or impact your life.

5–8 POINTS = No Priority Prescription: Don't discount this nutritional concern, even if you have very few symptoms. Somebody with a diagnosis of (for example) diabetes might not have any or many symptoms because he or she is in treatment and on medication, but diabetes is a serious disease and may still be the place you should start.

YOUR FREQUENTLY ASKED QUESTIONS— AND SOME ANSWERS

Our community is dynamic and curious and smart, and you always have questions that impress and challenge and delight me. I love that you are so curious! I want to answer all of them, so in this chapter I have anticipated as many as I can, based on those asked me over the years. And if your question isn't here, check my website, where I continually engage with my community to keep everybody inspired and on track (www.hayliepomroy.com). Your question may be there, or you can even ask me yourself.

When I go through the Self-Discovery Zones in this chapter, I see a lot of crossover in symptoms. How can the same symptom be an indication of multiple issues?

Multiple issues in one complex biodynamic body do have crossover symptoms. Every issue and imbalance I talk about is linked to other imbalances. I personally resonate strongly with three out of these seven chapters with some of my symptoms, so I rotate those three styles of eating. Each symptom gives a clue, but it's the symptom profile in total that gives us the answer. It's the combination of symptoms in total that points to a direction for repair. For a period of time, focus your efforts on targeted metabolic pathways with strategic food plans to disrupt the imbalance and promote a healthier rebalancing.

Sometimes I feel too overwhelmed to follow a plan. Are there simpler ways to benefit?

Absolutely. Here are some ways to dip a toe in the water rather than leaping in headfirst:

- Find the list of power foods for your prescription, make a copy, keep it with you, and eat those foods as often as you can. This is a simple way to make progress.

- Make strategic dinners—just make dinners that support cholesterol, or mood, or hormone, or autoimmune, or whatever prescription you want to work on, but don't worry about other meals just yet.

- Pick one simple rule and practice that. For example, in the autoimmune chapter (Chapter 11), part of the prescription is to eat fruit alone, always away from other foods. You could just start with that one thing.

- You could incorporate the lifestyle changes if you aren't ready to change your food, such as the targeted exercise or scheduling a massage or a laughing/joy session.

- You could follow the Guidelines for the General Rx (Chapter 4) to prepare yourself for more structure later. For example, master eating within thirty minutes of waking. Just work on that.

Go at whatever pace is right for you. You are already perfect. You don't need to try so hard to become perfect. Every small change can make a huge difference!

I took the Self-Assessment Questionnaire (page 44) and I don't want to do the program my body recommends I do first. Is there another approach? Can I start with a different plan?

Great question! Most of us can benefit from any of these plans. Here are some additional ideas for selecting the plan you want to begin with or the plan you want to do next. Ask yourself these questions:

- Which issues are bothering me the most?

- Which issue is most negatively impacting my life right now?

- Which issue is the most medically urgent?

- Which issue is my doctor most concerned about?

- Which Power Foods list is the most appealing to me?

- Which recipes look the best to me?

- Which plan looks like it will fit my current lifestyle best?

Although some doctors, especially functional medicine doctors, want to treat the whispers first—such as digestion—this might or might not be the best approach for you. Sometimes, you need to address the screaming baby in the corner or the screaming man on the rooftop. If a less than perfect childhood landed you in jail as a forty-year-old, you can't go back and heal your childhood wounds until you find a way to be bailed out! Sometimes people are so far down the path that they have to start right where they are at. Get to the root of the big issue, then go back and look at how it started and address that.

But maybe you'd rather start at the beginning and work your way through. That's fine, too. Whispers can be the building blocks for dysfunction, so if you dismantle those first, you can topple the whole dysfunctional structure. If you want to start with digestion, then move on to energy, then move on to hormones, and work your way through this book in order, that's also a great approach and will create a solid foundation for health, mopping up issues as you go like so much dirt on the kitchen floor. By the time you get to the end of the book, you'll be feeling fantastic.

If you begin by addressing the whisper, and it doesn't calm the scream within the first thirty days, then you need to address the scream instead.

If your body's not screaming, you can play around a bit and see what calls out to you. Maybe you really like the foods on one of the lists. Look through and see. Maybe one of the lists has foods that you really don't like. So start elsewhere. Sometimes, when people are making big changes to a healthy diet (such as if you tend to eat a lot of processed food), it's easier to start with healthy foods you like and, as your palate adjusts, you will find you enjoy foods you never thought you would later on in your dietary progression.

This book lays out seven of the custom nutrition plans I use in my clinic every day. You can't pick a wrong plan to start with, so go with what feels right and what you most want to deal with up front. Then move on from there. You can do this! The most important thing is to remember that you are a multidimensional, dynamic body. Remain curious!

How do I incorporate my nutritional prescription with FMD and/or The Burn?

My *Fast Metabolism Diet* (FMD) is a holistic plan to maximize the metabolic pathways that burn fat for fuel. It is a strategic, twenty-eight-day diet that can be repeated endlessly, cycling between rest and restoration, build and repair, continuously nurturing an umbrella of metabolic pathways. We even have a quiz in the Self-Discovery Zone on our website (www.hayliepomroy .com) that helps you identify if one of the three phases in the Fast Metabolism Diet needs additional nurturing and repair. So in my clinical practice, we "program hop" quite a bit. If difficulty losing weight is an overriding symptom, I oftentimes have an individual do a twenty-eight-day Fast Metabolism Diet push before we go into one of the food prescriptions. If weight is not an issue, we go directly into the food prescriptions. If an individual is dealing with diabetes or autoimmune disorders, oftentimes we do the food prescription first, cycling in a twenty-eight-day total body metabolic repair on the Fast Metabolism Diet two to four times a year.

On the other hand, *The Burn* consists of strategic three-, five-, and ten-day plans that can be repeated up to three times in a row. Clinically, I employ these nutrition plans when I find we have hit a plateau, not only on the scale but as a plateau in symptom relief. Let's say for example an individual is working on an autoimmune disorder and we want to strategically push GI repair. I will employ five to fifteen days of the D-Burn, right in the middle of our autoimmune prescription. In addition, if you take the Burn Quiz (you can also find this in the Self-Discovery Zone at www.hayliepomroy.com) and one of them stands out as being beneficial, you can simply layer its Success Boosters or the tea right on top of your current food prescription. It is not uncommon that I have individuals dealing with hormones or mood disorders on our H-Burn tea, or that I have individuals dealing with IBS and GI issues employing the Success Boosters on the D-Burn. All of these are tools to give your body what it's asking for.

I'm confused about portion sizes. How do I know how much to eat of any given food?

I put portions right at the top of each category of food on the Foundational Foods List. Although this is not a plan designed for weight loss necessarily, these are healthy portions that provide enough nutrients for metabolic repair. For example, vegetables are unlimited, a serving of fruit is 1 cup or 1 piece, and a serving of animal protein is 4 ounces of meat, or 6 ounces of fish, or 2 eggs. In my book *The Fast Metabolism Diet*, serving sizes were different depending on how much weight you had to lose, but the serving sizes in this book are general guidelines that apply to everyone in all situations. If you feel as if the portion sizes are too small or you need more food, first increase your vegetable portion. If this doesn't seem enough or if you have a high activity level, you can also increase your portion by an additional 50 percent to 6 ounces of meat, 9 ounces of fish, or 3 eggs.

For your easy reference, here is a chart showing portion sizes for all food groups:

FOOD CATEGORY	SERVING SIZE
Vegetables	Unlimited
Fruits	1 cup or 1 piece
COMPLEX CARBS	
Grains	1 cup cooked
Crackers/pretzels	1 ounce
Bread/tortilla	1 slice/1 tortilla
Bagel	½ bagel
ANIMAL PROTEIN	
Meat	4 ounces raw
Fish	6 ounces raw
Eggs	2 eggs
VEGETARIAN PROTEIN	
Legumes/cooked mushrooms	½ cup
Grains	½ cup
Nuts	¼ cup
HEALTHY FATS	
Almond milk	1 cup
Hummus/guacamole	⅓ cup
Avocado	½ avocado
Raw nuts and seeds	¼ cup
Dressing	3 tablespoons
Oil	2 tablespoons
Raw nut and seed butters	2 tablespoons
Herbs, spices, and condiments	Unlimited

How strict is the Foundational Foods List? Can I eat foods that aren't on it once in a while?

I've created this list for its ability to encourage repair. I find that to make a clinical change, when people apply their prescription even 75 percent of the time, it typically materializes. There is real value in recognizing that the more support you give yourself, though, the more symptom regression you will experience. But every little bit helps.

What about alcohol, sugar, and other treats that aren't on the Foundational Foods List, like french fries? Can I have those once in a while?

I monitor my health with my doctors fairly carefully, and I have a lot of demands on my body. For this reason, I feel the effects fairly quickly when I add these things to my life. I have to admit they have touched my lips, but I am quick to feel the adverse effects. Remain curious and give your body plenty of time to heal without these indulgences. Then, be acutely aware of what happens to your body when you do introduce them. The one exception is this: you will *never hear me say* that a soda, or pop, or Coke, or whatever you want to call it is not a big deal once in a while. It is a big deal, and I believe soda should never be part of anyone's diet.

Do I have to use fresh produce, or can I use frozen?

Many of my clients have tremendous success with freezing their own fresh vegetables, using commercially frozen, or even using canned. What's more important is that you strive for organic whenever possible.

Does everything have to be organic?

No, but whatever toxins you put into your body, your body has no choice but to deal with, and that takes time, energy, and effort. The cleaner the environment you can provide for the body—food, air, water, and cleaning products—the less work, time, and, effort the body has to spend eliminating those from your system. This means it can spend that much more work, time, and effort healing you.

You don't really say much about wheat or gluten in this book. Can I have wheat or gluten?

You will notice that, with the exception of sprouted grains, spelt, and Kamut, wheat and grains containing gluten are not a part of the Foundational Foods List. If you know you have celiac disease or you believe you have a sensitivity to wheat or gluten, or feel that it is a trigger for metabolic imbalance for you, make sure to avoid it, and that includes gluten-containing sprouted grains, spelt, and Kamut. Stick to non-gluten grains like quinoa, teff, buckwheat, millet, amaranth, and certified gluten-free oats. Even if you don't have a gluten intolerance, I still recommend that you stick to sprouted grains and more ancient forms of grain like quinoa, spelt, and Kamut rather than processed modern wheat.

What about dairy? I thought dairy was healthy. Why aren't there any dairy products on the Foundational Foods List?

In my twenty plus years of clinical experience, with the exception of some fertility issues, I haven't typically used dairy as a cornerstone for repair. When working on metabolic pathways, we have to be strategic with our micronutrients in any given food. Since many people don't respond well to dairy, we leave it out of these particular nutritional prescriptions.

I noticed corn and potatoes aren't on the Foundational Foods List. Does that mean I can't eat corn on the cob or a baked potato, or (gasp!) tortilla chips or potato chips? Even if they are baked?

Corn and potatoes are typically not nutrient-dense. They have a high carbohydrate content, and they contain a lot of "fluff" as far as giving the body quick fuel, yet they don't provide the body with building blocks for repair. For this reason, they tend to get in the way of what we're trying to do with the metabolism. I find they are more likely to provide the body with crisis fuel, rather than strategic restorative fuel, so we skip them for now. There are more interesting foods for you to discover and nosh!

What if food I thought was healthy isn't on the Foundational Foods List? For example, grapes or bananas. Does that mean I can't eat them?

The foods on the Foundational Foods List are not chosen for what they don't contain. I chose them for what they *do* contain. Each was selected for its healing properties, so some "healthy foods" just didn't make the list. But as your prescription sets in and begins to work its magic, you will find that as a community, we love all food as long as it can legally and ethically bear that name (i.e., it was once alive and came from the earth, water, or sky).

Why are some foods in a particular food category in The Fast Metabolism Diet, *but in a different category in this book?*

Oh, you savvy and observant readers! Good job spotting this. When I create a meal map for a client, I work strategically to manipulate blood sugar, enzymatic production, and micronutrient assimilation, and I am also attempting to bring about therapeutic levels of strategic nutrients for repair. When I create a meal map and I make categories for foods in order to fill that meal map, I put them into categories specifically for the jobs I want them to do. So, yes, the food scientist in me knows that tomatoes are technically a fruit, but in some cases, I use them as a vegetable. In *Fast Metabolism Diet*, for example, I used tomatoes for their lycopene and fiber value, and for that particular purpose, I needed them to count as a vegetable. In this book, however, and for our specific purposes here, tomatoes are valuable for their carbohydrates and natural sugar content. As another example, legumes like pinto beans, black beans, and chickpeas are proteins in *Fast Metabolism Diet*, but for our purposes here they count as complex carbohydrates. In reality, they are both complex carbs and proteins, but again, my use is highly strategic, so please follow the categories as written that are relevant to the plan you are currently using.

Nuts and seeds are listed as both a protein and a healthy fat. If you want raw nuts for protein, does that mean you can have an additional healthy fat, if the prescription calls for a protein and a healthy fat in a meal?

No, you could have additional protein because the protein content is comparatively low in nuts, but you cannot do an additional fat because the fat content of the nuts is high. Nuts can act as either/or when the meal calls for a protein or a fat because they contain both macronutrients. But because they contain adequate fat, you don't need to add more. Because they have lower protein, you can add lean protein when called for in a meal map or recipe.

Other books say no rice vinegar, but the Foundational Foods List says to use any vinegar. Is rice vinegar okay now? As long as it doesn't have added sugar?

Any vinegar is fine as long as there is no sugar added. But remember, there is no rice allowed for those dealing with the autoimmune prescription, and do pay attention to the rice vinegar you purchase, because many brands of that type in particular tend to have added sugar.

What do you consider to be "lean" meat? What percentage of fat is lean, such as with ground beef?

I don't mind if you purchase any kind of ground beef—just drain off the fat. Lean meat doesn't include pork bacon or pork sausage, or shrimp or lamb, and if you do have a steak, trim off the obvious fat. Otherwise, most fresh meat counts as lean.

How is the GI chapter different from the D-Burn?

The D-Burn is strategic in helping your body break through a plateau. It only lasts for five days. We go much deeper in the GI prescription in this book, in repairing and regenerating tissue and re-inoculating the microbiome. The GI chapter is a long-term repair solution.

How is the PMS, Perimenopause, Menopause, and Manopause chapter different from the H-Burn?

The H-Burn is strategically designed to dislodge a barrier to success, and it only lasts for ten days. It is a short-term blast to your hormones. The hormone-related chapter in this book (Chapter 7) is a long-term healing prescription. Many of the components of the H-Burn, such as the tea, soup, and the Success Boosters, can be layered into the comprehensive hormonal prescription chapter in this book with great success, if you desire to do so.

How do I ask for medical tests?

Earlier in this book I discussed doctors and how to talk to them, as well as what to ask for and how to advocate for yourself. This can be challenging, for many reasons. Some doctors don't see the need for these tests. Some don't like to be told to do things they think a patient "found on the Internet" (and this happens a lot). Also, they don't want to leave you strapped with excessive bills, and insurance companies demand reasons for tests before they will cover them. For all these reasons, I give you a little more help.

For instance, I tell you frequently to put your lab requests in writing, along with those symptoms you defined in the Self-Discovery Zones. But how do you do that? I help my clients with this by providing them with letter samples that they can use. On pages 258–259 is an example of one such letter.

Adapt this to your own situation, print it out, and give it to your doctor. Don't put on pressure or assume you will get an unfriendly response. Be casual and friendly, and say something like, "I printed this out for you, but I want to go over a few things."

Here are some things to notice about this letter:

- It is polite, clear, and simple, with bulleted lists of symptoms and text that are easy to see and read without taking too much time.

- It uses medical terms like dysmenorrhea (which means painful menstruation) to make it easier for a doctor to justify tests without translating. If you don't know the medical term, you don't need to use it, but if you do, go for it.

Dear Dr. Sanders:

I am having some health issues that are very concerning to me. In addition to the normal labs we would run at this visit, can we please run some diagnostics, so that we can help define what's going on with me? The reason I am requesting these is because I am experiencing:

- Hair loss and thinning at the crown. This is not normal for me.
- Chin acne
- Unexplained rapid weight gain (my activity and caloric intake have not varied)
- Extreme breast tenderness

Also please note that:

- I have a previous diagnosis of adenomyosis
- I have a positive gene for Alzheimer's and heart disease (APOE-e4) and my mother already suffers from dementia, with onset in her late 60s.
- My younger sister suffered a heart attack at age 47 and my mother suffered a heart attack at age 70.
- I am 49 and premenopausal.

Because of rapid weight gain, I would like to run:

- Hemoglobin A1
- Fasting glucose (blood sugar)
- Fasting insulin

Because of hair loss and weight gain, I would like to run:

- TSH
- T3/T4 free and uptake

Because of age and cardiovascular risk, I would like to run:

- CRP
- Lipid panel

Because of dysmenorrhea and age, I would like to run:

- E2
- FSH
- LH
- Progesterone
- Testosterone free and total

Thank you for your time.
Sincerely,

- It doesn't contain any self-diagnosis, only actual previous diagnoses and family history. Beyond that, it asks for tests so the *doctor* can make the diagnosis, which is, after all the doctor's job.

- It is not wishy-washy. It is your right to ask for and receive lab tests (even if it isn't necessarily your right for insurance to pay for them all—but you might as well try!).

HERE'S TO A NEW YOU

I want to encourage you in your new life. I want you to feel comfortable in your new role as . . . well, what was once called a "health nut" but what is now so necessary for survival in our modern world. Instead, let's call you the captain of your own team.

Are you ready to move forward with your life, Captain? That means being proactive. That means never again standing back and letting other people control your choices and what you do. That means if your family eats at a restaurant every Friday night, but there is really nothing you can eat there to maintain and build your health, you go out and do some research and find a better restaurant. Or, you change the plan and start a family potluck at home, with everybody contributing something that can make you all feel stronger, better, and healthier.

That means researching in your community where you can buy food. What are the best grocery stores? Where are the best cafes? Who is serving food that builds health and which places do you want to avoid? You might even find that your social circles change a bit. Best friends are forever, but that doesn't mean you can't make new friends who fuel your good habits and support and encourage you as you make changes and gain more and more health.

And stay curious! Find new websites, and apps, and online food sources that serve you. Embrace cooking. Bring your own dishes to dinner parties, so you can eat to treat while being social and having fun. This might mean asking for gluten-free communion wafers, if that's what you need. It means getting together with friends to laugh and talk, and walk and share. Paint or go to a museum or concert together. Don't gorge on pizza or binge on margaritas (although there is a place for those things . . . but maybe they don't have to be the central part of your social life).

Finally, be part of our community. I've got a ton of online resources, from communities and Q&As, recipes, and shared experiences, and even products that make life easier. My community is a safe place designed to explore the "you" in your health.

So, let me feed you. With information. With hope. With acceptance. And with ideas for better health. Be patient with yourself. Remember, if a car is speeding down the road in the wrong direction, you can't do a U-turn at 100 miles per hour. First, you understand that you don't have to go the wrong way; then you slow down and look for when it's safe to turn. Then and only then do you make the actual turn and start going in the right direction.

I feel that I am living a health victory, but that victory didn't happen overnight, and it's not really over. When I get nervous, I bake. You, too, can find that thing that helps you relax. A health food store feels like a sanctuary for me. Find that place that feels like a sanctuary to you. Clean organic food provides me with comfort and solace. It can do the same for you. There was a time when I felt I had lost control of my own metabolic pathways. I knew I needed the right prescription—and you know when you need it, too. That prescription is food. It has given me the privilege to break bread with you. I am so grateful for that.

Acknowledgments

I owe so much to so many. There will never be enough ways to say thank you. But let me try.

Ode to Alex Glass, the best literary agent that ever was! Without you none of this would be possible. Your efforts, conviction, and friendship have allowed me to manifest so many personal dreams and help so many people in my life's work. You are a rock star!

I am so grateful to Crown/Harmony Books, the best literary partners any author could ever ask for. Heather Jackson, you hold my mission so respectfully and thoughtfully as if it's your own, then you make every single part of it better—that is talent! Diana Baroni, Maya Mavjee, Aaron Wehner, Tammy Blake, Christina Foxley, Julie Cepler, Luisa Francavilla, Henri Clinch (my partner in App crime) and Tina Constable you all created this and your work will save lives and make a lasting impact.

Eve Adamson, you get me and that is both fun and a bit scary! Melanie Parish, your love and business guidance have been invaluable. Bob Marty, thank you for taking us to unbelievable Public Television success; and Marc Chamlin, your legal advice is almost as profound as your personal advice. To Kym, Leilani, Keyanna, John, Carol, Andrew, Dominique, and the HPG Team you are changing lives and touching hearts and your "all in" tireless spirit makes everything possible. I cherish you. To my beloved community, clients, and virtual clients: thank you for sharing your journey and allowing me to walk with you on my own. You inspire me.

I want to say a heartfelt thank-you to the amazing doctors and practitioners who joined my team to ensure my own health: Dr. Richard Hawkins,

Dr. Karo Arzoo, Dr. Ahdoot, Dr. Gerald McIntosh, Beth Fondy, Dr. Christine Szeto, and Dr. Jackie Fields.

I am so grateful to my mom and dad, my sisters and sisters-in-law, my brother outlaws, my nieces and nephews, my crazy kids, and my never-wavering, solid-as-a-rock husband who thinks everything I write is perfect (may he be right always.) I love you all with all of my heart.

—Haylie Pomroy

Appendix

A. Foundational Foods List

These are the foods that will form the foundation of your daily diet. They can be eaten in any of the plans to help you follow your specific nutritional prescriptions. Even if you have none of the health issues discussed in this book, and just want a healthy foundation for eating, choose from this list. It is your go-to source for health.

VEGETABLES

SERVING SIZE: UNLIMITED

Alfalfa sprouts

Artichokes—all types, fresh, frozen, jarred, or canned without additives, not marinated. Artichokes and water should be the only ingredients stated on package.

Arugula

Asparagus

Bamboo shoots

Beans—green, yellow wax, haricots verts

Bean sprouts

Beets—fresh or canned, no sugar added

Beets—greens and bulbs

Bok choy

Broccoli

Broccolini

Brussels sprouts

Cabbage—all types, including fermented/cultured, such as sauerkraut and kimchi

Carrots

Cauliflower

Celery—including leaves

Chicory—especially curly endive

Collard greens

Cucumbers—all types

Cultured/fermented veggies—all types, such as sauerkraut, kimchi, and cultured pickles

Daikon (white radish)

Dandelion greens

Eggplant

Endive

Fennel

Frisée
Hearts of palm
Jícama
Kale
Leafy greens (mixed)
Leeks
Lettuces—all types except iceberg
Mushrooms
Mustard greens
Okra
Onions—red, yellow, green (scallions)
Parsnips
Peppers—sweet and hot: Anaheim, banana, cherry, habanero, jalapeño, pepperoncini, poblano, and serrano chiles; bell, Italian frying, pimiento, sweet peppers (Note: all peppers, including spices from chiles, such as red pepper flakes and cayenne, are to be avoided when on the autoimmune prescription)

Pumpkin
Radishes
Rhubarb
Rutabaga
Sea vegetable/seaweeds—dulse, hijiki, kelp, kombu, nori
Shallots
Snow peas
Spinach
Spirulina (type of algae)
Sprouts—all types
Summer squash— yellow, zucchini
Swiss chard
Turnips
Watercress
Winter squash—acorn, butternut, delicata, pumpkin, spaghetti squash

FRUITS

Note: All fruits and vegetables can be fresh or frozen, unless otherwise noted.

SERVING SIZE: 1 CUP OR 1 PIECE

Low glycemic fruits (0–49)

Apples—all types
Blackberries
Blueberries
Cherries
Goji berries
Grapefruit
Kumquats
Lemons
Limes
Loganberries

Mulberries
Oranges
Peaches
Pears—all types
Plums
Prickly pears
Prunes
Strawberries
Tomatoes (for our purposes, tomatoes are fruit, not vegetable)

High glycemic fruits (50–100)

Apricots
Cantaloupe
Clementine
Cranberries
Figs—fresh only
Guavas
Honeydew melon
Kiwi

Mangos
Nectarines
Papayas
Pineapple
Pomegranates
Raspberries
Tangerines
Watermelon

COMPLEX CARBS

SERVING SIZE: 1 CUP COOKED GRAIN; ½ CUP COOKED LEGUMES; 1 OUNCE CRACKERS OR PRETZELS; 1 SLICE BREAD; 1 TORTILLA; ½ BAGEL; 1 MEDIUM SWEET POTATO

Amaranth

Barley—black or white

Beans/legumes—white, black, kidney, lima, pinto, adzuki; no peanuts, peas or soybeans

Brown rice pasta

Buckwheat flour

Kamut flour/bagels

Freekah (a green wheat that is roasted; considered an "ancient grain")

Millet

Nut flours

Oats/oatmeal

Quinoa

Rice—brown, black, red, wild

Rye flour

Sorghum

Spelt—pasta, pretzels, tortillas

Sprouted-grain bagels, breads, tortillas

Sweet potatoes/yams (for our purposes, sweet potatoes and yams are complex carbs, not vegetables)

Tapioca, as a thickener in recipes (not the pudding with added sugar)

Teff

Wheat grass (serving size one shot)

PROTEINS

ANIMAL PROTEIN

SERVING SIZE: 4 OUNCES MEAT OR 6 OUNCES FISH

Beef—all lean cuts, lean ground meat, rump roast

Buffalo

Calamari

Caviar

Chicken

Clams

Corned beef

Crabmeat

Cured lean meats—prosciutto, black forest ham, smoked ham (only if nitrate free)

Deli meats—turkey, chicken, roast beef (only if nitrate free)

Eggs, whole, any size (2 eggs make a serving)

Fish—wild-caught, any types, especially cod, dory, flounder, haddock, halibut, herring, mackerel, pollock, sardines, sea bass, skate, sole, and trout (avoid bottom feeders, which tend to be more polluted, such as tilapia, grouper, and catfish)

Game—venison, elk, pheasant, etc.

Guinea fowl

Jerky—beef, buffalo, turkey, elk, ostrich

Lamb

Lobster

Mussels

Organ meats—chicken liver or gizzards, beef liver or heart, sweetbreads, kidneys, etc.

Oysters, fresh, raw or cooked; or packaged, packed in water

Pork—tenderloin, loin roast, chops

Rabbit

Salmon—smoked, fresh, frozen, or canned

Scallops

Shrimp

Tuna—fresh, frozen, or canned

Turkey

VEGETARIAN PROTEIN

SERVING SIZE: 1/2 CUP COOKED LEGUMES/COOKED MUSHROOMS; 1/2 CUP COOKED
GRAINS; 1/4 CUP RAW NUTS

Note: Some items on this list also appear on other lists, such as the Complex Carbs, Vegetables, or Healthy Fats lists. These foods can be used for either purpose in your meal map, but serving sizes will vary depending on how you are using them.

Almond cheese/almond flour

Beans/legumes—white, black, pinto, chickpeas, lentils, adzuki, etc.—all *except* peanuts, peas, or soybeans

Mushrooms

Nuts and seeds—raw only, all types (almond, Brazil, chia, pecan, pumpkin, sesame, walnuts, etc.), including their butters

Oat bran

Quinoa

Rye berries

Wild rice

HEALTHY FATS

SERVING SIZE: 1 CUP NUT MILKS; 1/4 CUP RAW NUTS AND SEEDS OR SHREDDED
COCONUT; 1/4 CUP OLIVES; 3 TABLESPOONS DRESSING; 2 TABLESPOONS OIL;
2 TABLESPOONS RAW NUT OR SEED BUTTERS

Almond milk

Avocado—1/2 medium

Cashew milk

Coconut

Coconut milk

Coconut oil

Flaxseed

Grapeseed oil

Hummus (1/3 cup)

Mayonnaise—safflower oil based

Olive oil

Olives

Nuts and seeds—raw only, all types (almond, Brazil, chia, pumpkin, sesame, walnuts, etc.), including their butters

Sesame oil

Tahini (sesame butter)

HERBS, SPICES, CONDIMENTS, AND MISCELLANEOUS FOODS

SERVING SIZE: UNLIMITED

Agar

Apple cider vinegar

Arrowroot powder

Black pepper

Broths and stocks, homemade or natural/sugar-free—beef, chicken, vegetable, turkey

Cacao powder, raw

Chili powder

Chives

Coconut aminos

Dried or fresh herbs—basil, bay leaf, celery seed, dill, mint, oregano, parsley, rosemary, tarragon, thyme (Note: all peppers, including spices from chiles, such as red pepper flakes and cayenne, are to be avoided when on the autoimmune prescription)

Garlic—fresh, and garlic powder

Ginger, fresh or ground

Horseradish, fresh or jarred

Lemon peel, lemon verbena leaves

Lime peel

Mustard—all types

Nutritional yeast

Pickles

Salsa, including fermented

Sea salt

Sesame seeds

Spices—cinnamon, coriander, cumin, turmeric, nutmeg

Spices from peppers—cayenne pepper, chili powder, red pepper flakes, paprika, etc.

Sweeteners—pure stevia or birch-based xylitol

Tabasco

Tamari

Vanilla extract

Vinegars—any type (including coconut vinegar and rice vinegar as long as it doesn't contain added sugar)

Xanthan gum (non-corn based)

B. Top 20 Power Foods for GI Repair

Basil

Carrots

Celery

Coconut oil

Cultured/fermented cabbage (such as kimchi and sauerkraut)

Fennel

Green apples

Green beans

Lentils (ideally sprouted)

Mint

Pears

Pine nuts

Prunes

Raw pumpkin seeds

Red cabbage

Rosemary

Salmon

Sweet potatoes

Zucchini

C. Top 20 Power Foods for Energy Repair

Asparagus

Brussels sprouts

Cantaloupe

Cauliflower

Celery

Chiles

Coconut oil

Cucumbers

Eggs

Fish—wild-caught, except tilapia, grouper, or catfish

Ginger, fresh or ground

Grapefruit

Lemons

Lentils

Meats—all lean types

Nuts, raw

Oatmeal

Quinoa

Raspberries

Spinach

D. Top 20 Power Foods for Hormone Repair

Apples

Avocados

Beets

Black pepper

Blueberries

Broccoli

Cabbage

Cinnamon

Eggs, whole (not just whites), organic

Flaxseed

Garlic

Ginger, fresh or ground

Legumes

Olive oil

Oranges

Pineapples

Nuts, raw

Sweet potatoes

Turmeric

Salmon, wild-caught

E. Top 20 Power Foods for Cholesterol Metabolism Repair

Avocados

Green beans

Berries, such as raspberries, blueberries, blackberries

Carrots

Fish—any kind

Garlic

Legumes—lentils, black beans, kidney beans, chickpeas

Mushrooms

Oats

Onions

Oranges

Pears

Pork—lean and nitrite free

Prunes

Radishes

Rosemary

Sardines

Spinach

Tomatoes

Walnuts

F. Top 20 Power Foods for Mood and Cognition Repair

Apricots

Beef liver (organic only)

Broccoli

Cantaloupe

Carrots

Cashews

Chickpeas

Collard greens

Cultured (fermented) veggies

Lima beans

Mackerel

Oranges

Oysters

Peaches

Pumpkin

Salmon

Sardines

Spinach

Turkey

Walnuts

G. Top 20 Power Foods for Blood Sugar Repair

Artichokes

Avocados

Beef (grass-fed)

Bell peppers

Cauliflower

Chia seeds

Coconut milk

Dark leafy greens, especially dandelion greens and spinach

Eggplant

Fresh herbs, especially parsley, rosemary, and chives

Garlic

Green beans

Lettuce

Nuts, raw—all types

Olives

Onions

Turkey (organic)

Vinegar—all types without added sugar

Warming spices like chili powder, cayenne pepper, cinnamon, and turmeric

Zucchini

H. Top 20 Power Foods for Immune Repair

Apricots

Arugula

Asparagus

Beef liver (organic)

Blueberries

Brussels sprouts

Butternut squash

Cauliflower

Celery

Cranberries

Cucumbers

Garlic

Jícama

Olives

Radishes

Sardines

Sprouted adzuki beans

Sweet potatoes

Turkey

Watermelon

I. Avoid Autoimmunity Anti-power Foods

Although the foods on this list are generally considered nutritious, they can be triggers for autoimmunity. If this is your challenge, temporarily cross these foods off your Foundational Foods List.

Almonds

Cherries

Chiles and peppers, including all sweet and hot chiles and peppers like bell, banana, frying peppers, jalapeños, pimientos, and habanero; as well as spices made from peppers, like paprika and cayenne (black pepper is okay)

Eggplant

Eggs

Goji berries

White potatoes (sweet potatoes are okay)

Rice

Sprouted grain, spelt, and Kamut (only if you have celiac disease or gluten intolerance)

Tomatillos

Tomatoes

Anyone with an autoimmune disorder must carefully read ingredients and look for hidden gluten, dairy, corn, rice, potatoes, and soy products. These are common triggers for autoimmunity, and although you won't be intentionally eating them because they aren't on your Foundational Foods List, they are commonly hidden in prepared foods. Products labeled "gluten-free" are not necessarily safe, as they often contain dairy, corn, rice, potatoes, or soy.

References

Abu Shakra, M., D. Buskila, M. Ehrenfeld, K. Conrad, and Y. Shoenfeld. "Cancer and Autoimmunity: Autoimmune and Rheumatic Features in Patients with Malignancies." *Annals of the Rheumatic Diseases* 60, no. 5 (January 2001): 433–41.

Adiels, M., et al. "Liver, Belly Fat May Identify High Risks of Heart Disease in Obese People." American Heart Association website posting, July 2011; http://newsroom.heart.org/news/1386.

Alcock, J., C. C. Maley, and C. A. Aktipis. "Is Eating Behavior Manipulated by the Gastrointestinal Microbiota? Evolutionary Pressures and Potential Mechanisms." *Bioessays* 36 (August 2014): 1–10.

Anathaswamy, A. "Fecal Transplant Eases Symptoms of Parkinson's." *New Scientist* 106 (January 19, 2011): S352.

Bell, J. A., M. Kivimaki, and M. Hamer. "Metabolically Healthy Obesity and Risk of Incident Type 2 Diabetes: A Meta-analysis of Prospective Cohort Studies." *Obesity Reviews* 15, no. 6 (June 2014): 504–15; http://onlinelibrary.wiley.com/enhanced/doi/10.1111/obr.12157/.

Bergström, J., and E. Hultman. "Nutrition for Maximal Sports Performance." *Journal of the American Medical Association* 9 (1972): 999–1006.

Bes-Rastrollo, M., et al. "Prospective Study of Nut Consumption, Long-term Weight Change, and Obesity Risk in Women. *American Journal of Clinical Nutrition* 89, no. 6 (April 2009): 1913–19.

Bloom, D. E., et al. *The Global Economic Burden of Non-communicable Diseases*, A report by the World Economic Forum and the Harvard School of Public Health, September 2011. http://www3.weforum.org/docs/WEF_Harvard_HE_GlobalEconomicBurdenNonCommunicableDiseases_2011.pdf.

Bostrom, P., et al. "A PGC1-a-dependent Myokine that Drives Brown-fat-like Development of White Fat and Thermogenesis." *Nature* 481 (January 2012): 463–68.

Bovet, P., D. Faeh, G. Madeleine, B. Viswanathan, and F. Paccaud. "Decrease in Blood Triglycerides Associated with the Consumption of Eggs of Hens Fed with Food Supplemented with Fish Oil." *Nutrition, Metabolism, and Cardiovascular Diseases* 17, no. 4 (May 2007): 280–87.

Brookes, L. "Significant New Definitions, Publications, Risks, Benefits: American Heart Association and National Heart, Lung and Blood Institute Update ATP III Definition of Metabolic Syndrome," from *Hypertension Highlights*, a Medscape Cardiology article. http://www.medscape.org/viewarticle/514644.

Brotherhood, J. R. "Nutrition and Sports Performance." *Sports Medicine* 1, no. 5 (September 1984): 350–89.

Bundy, R., A. F. Walker, R. W. Middleton, and J. Booth. "Turmeric Extract May Improve Irritable Bowel Syndrome Symptomology in Otherwise Healthy Adults: A Pilot Study." *Journal of Alternative and Complementary Medicine* 10, no. 6 (December 2004): 1015–18.

Burke, L. M. "Caffeine and Sports Performance." *Applied Physiology, Nutrition, and Metabolism* 33, no. 6 (July 2008): 1319–34.

Burton-Freeman, B. M., et al. "Whole Food versus Supplement: Comparing the Clinical Evidence of Tomato Intake and Lycopene Supplementation on Cardiovascular Risk Factors," *Advances in Nutrition* 5 (2014): 457–85.

Caforio, A. L. P., et al. "Evidence from Family Studies for Autoimmunity in Dilated Cardiomyopathy." *The Lancet* 344, no. 8925 (September 1994): 773–77.

Camilleri, M. "Serotonin in the Gastrointestinal Tract." *Current Opinion in Endocrinology, Diabetes and Obesity* 16, no. 1 (February 2010): 53–59.

Campbell, K. L., et al. "Reduced-Calorie Dietary Weight Loss, Exercise, and Sex Hormones in Postmenopausal Women: Randomized Controlled Trial." *Journal of Clinical Oncology* 30, no. 10 (July 2012): 2314–26.

Canavan, C., J. West, and T. Card. "The Epidemiology of Irritable Bowel Syndrome." *Clinical Epidemiology* 6 (2014): 71–80.

Castro, C., and M. Gourley. "Diagnostic Testing and Interpretation of Tests for Autoimmunity." *Journal of Allergy and Clinical Immunology* 125, no. 2 (January 2010): 238–47.

Centers for Disease Control and Prevention. "Chronic Diseases and Health Promotion." CDC website posting, July 2015; http://www.cdc.gov/chronicdisease/overview/.

Chambers, E. S., M. W. Bridge, and D. A. Jones. "Carbohydrate Sensing in the Human Mouth: Effects on Exercise Performance and Brain Activity." *Journal of Physiology* 587, no. 8 (April 2009): 1779–94.

Coppack, S. W., et al. "Adipose Tissue Metabolism in Obesity: Lipase Action in vivo Before and After a Mixed Meal." *Metabolism: Clinical and Experimental* 41, no. 3 (1992): 264–72.

Corthals, A. P. "Multiple Sclerosis Is Not a Disease of the Immune System." *Quarterly Review of Biology* 86, no. 4 (December 2011): 287–321.

David, L. A., et al. "Diet Rapidly and Reproducibly Alters the Human Gut Microbiome." *Nature* 505 (January 2014): 559–63.

Endocrine Society. "Studies on Metabolic Adaptation." *Endocrinology* 21 (2013).

Esposito, K., and D. Giugliano. "Obesity, the Metabolic Syndrome, and Sexual Dysfunction." *International Journal of Impotence Research* 17 (May 2005): 391–98.

Esposito, K., et al. "Effect of Lifestyle Changes on Erectile Dysfunction in Obese Men: A Randomized Controlled Trial." *Journal of the American Medical Association* 291, no. 24 (June 2004): 2978–84.

Felger, J. C., and F. E. Lotrich. "Inflammatory Cytokines in Depression: Neurobiological Mechanisms and Therapeutic Implications." *Neuroscience* 246 (2013): 199–229.

Fernandez, M. L. "Rethinking Dietary Cholesterol." *Current Opinion in Clinical Nutrition and Metabolic Care* 15, no. 2 (March 2012): 117–21.

Ghadirian P., M. Jain, S. Ducic, B. Shatenstein, and R. Morisset. "Nutritional Factors in the Aetiology of Multiple Sclerosis: A Case-control Study in Montreal, Canada." *International Journal of Epidemiology* 27, no. 5 (February 1998): 845–52.

Goldstein, D. S. "Adrenal Responses to Stress." *Cellular and Molecular Neurobiology* 30, no. 8 (2010): 1433–40.

Gonzalez, A., et al. "The Mind-Body-Microbial Continuum." *Dialogues of Clinical Neuroscience* 13, no. 1 (2011): 55–62.

"Gut-Brain Connection." *The Sensitive Gut*, March 2012. http://www.health.harvard.edu/healthbeat/the-gut-brain-connection.

Hodes, G. E., et al. "Individual Differences in the Peripheral Immune System Promote Resilience versus Susceptibility to Social Stress." *CrossMark: Proceedings of the National Academy of Sciences of the United States of America* 111, no. 45 (November 2014): 16136–41.

Hunter, J. O. "Nutritional Factors in Inflammatory Bowel Disease." *European Journal of Gastroenterology and Hepatology* 10, no. 3 (March 1998): 235–37.

Hyman, Mark. "This Gut Condition Affects One in Six People—And Is Entirely Treatable." Drhyman.com blog, posted April 4, 2015; http://drhyman.com/blog/2015/04/09/this-gut-condition-affects-one-in-six-people-and-is-entirely-treatable/#close.

"Intestinal Cancer and Celiac Disease." National Foundation for Celiac Awareness website posting, 2015; http://www.celiaccentral.org/Celiac-Disease/Related-Conditions/Intestinal-Cancer/46/.

"Is the Effect of Aerobic Exercise on Cognition a Placebo Effect?" *PLoS ONE* (October 2014); http://journals.plos.org/plosone/article?id=10.1371/journal.pone .0109557.

Joseph, C. G., et al. "Association of the Autoimmune Disease Scleroderma with an Immunologic Response to Cancer." *Science* 343, no. 6167 (January 2014): 152–57.

Kaliman, P., et al. "Rapid Changes in Histone Deacetylases and Inflammatory Gene Expression in Expert Meditators." *International Society of Psychoneuroendocrinology* 40 (February 2014): 96–107.

Katcher, H. I., et al. "The Effects of a Whole Grain-enriched Hypocaloric Diet on Cardiovascular Disease Risk Factors in Men and Women with Metabolic Syndrome 1,2,3." *American Journal of Clinical Nutrition* 87, no. 1 (January 2008): 79–90.

Kaya, A., et al. "Autoantibodies in Heart Failure and Cardiac Dysfunction." *Circulation Research* 110 (2012): 145–58.

Khan, A., M. Safdar, M. M. Ali Khan, K. N. Khattak, and R. A. Anderson. "Cinnamon Improves Glucose and Lipids of People with Type 2 Diabetes." *Diabetes Care* 26, no. 12 (December 2003): 3215–18.

Koo, L. C. "The Use of Food to Treat and Prevent Disease in Chinese Culture." *Social Science & Medicine* 19, no. 9 (1984): 757–66.

Kostis, J. B., et al.,"Sexual Dysfunction and Cardiac Risk (the Second Princeton Consensus Conference)." *American Journal of Cardiology* 96, no. 2 (July 2005): 313–21.

Landsberg, L., et al. "Obesity-related Hypertension: Pathogenesis, Cardiovascular Risk, and Treatment—A Position Paper of the Obesity Society and the American Society of Hypertension." *Obesity* 21, no. 1 (January 2013): 8–24.

Larsen, S., et al. "The Effect of High-intensity Training on Mitochondrial Fat Oxidation in Skeletal Muscle and Subcutaneous Adipose Tissue." *Scandinavian Journal of Medicine & Science in Sports* 25, no. 1 (February 2015): e59–69.

Li, Y., et al. "Aerobic, Resistance and Combined Exercise Training on Arterial Stiffness in Normotensive and Hypertensive Adults: A Review." *European Journal of Sport Science* 15, no. 5 (September 2014): 443–57.

Luo, C., et al. "Nut Consumption and Risk of Type 2 Diabetes, Cardiovascular Disease, and All-cause Mortality: A Systematic Review and Meta-analysis." *American Journal of Clinical Nutrition* 100, no. 1 (May 2014): 256–69.

Ma, J., et al. "Sugar-sweetened Beverage Consumption Is Associated with Abdominal Fat Partitioning in Healthy Adults." *Journal of Nutrition* 144, no. 8 (August 2014): 1283–90.

McEwen, B. S. "Physiology and Neurobiology of Stress and Adaptation: Central Role of the Brain." *Physiological Reviews* 87, no. 3 (2007): 873–904.

McKeown, N. M., et al. "Whole-Grain Intake and Cereal Fiber Are Associated with Lower Abdominal Adiposity in Older Adults." *Journal of Nutrition* 139, no. 10 (October 2009): 1950–55.

Mercola, Joseph. "Butter Is Back—Processed Foods Are Identified as Real Culprits in Heart Disease." Mercola.com website, June 2014; http://articles.mercola.com/sites/articles/archive/2014/06/23/butter-trans-fat.aspx.

Mercola, Joseph. "How Stress Wreaks Havoc on Your Gut—and What to Do About It." Mercola.com website, April 2012; http://articles.mercola.com/sites/articles/archive/2012/04/09/chronic-stress-gut-effects.aspx.

Mercola, Joseph. "Mounting Evidence Pegs Broccoli as One of Nature's Most Health-Promoting Foods, Tackling Hypertension, Cancer, and More." Mercola.com website, September 2012; http://articles.mercola.com/sites/articles/archive/2012/09/23/broccoli-health-benefits.aspx.

Mizgier, M. L., M. Casas, A. Contreras-Ferrat, P. Llanos, and J. E. Galgani. "Potential Role of Skeletal Muscle Glucose Metabolism on the Regulation of Insulin Secretion." *Obesity Reviews* 15, no. 7 (July 2014): 587–97.

"Most Common OTC Medications." Dailyrx.com website posting, April 2014; http://www.dailyrx.com/over-counter-medications-most-common-us-include-cough-cold-and-allergy-otc-remedies.

National Heart, Lung, and Blood Institute. "What Is Metabolic Syndrome?" National Institutes of Health website posting, November 2011; http://www.nhlbi.nih.gov/health/health-topics/topics/ms.

Norris, V., G. Molina, and A. T. Gewirtz. "Hypothesis: Bacteria Control Host Appetites." *Journal of Bacteriology* 195, no. 3 (February 2013): 411–16.

Ornish, D., et al. "Can Lifestyle Changes Reverse Coronary Heart Disease? The Lifestyle Heart Trial." *The Lancet* 336, no. 8708 (July 1990): 129–33.

Pesta, D. H., S. S. Angadi, M. Burtscher, and C. K. Roberts. "The Effects of Caffeine, Nicotine, Ethanol, and Tetrahydrocannabinol on Exercise Performance." *Nutrition & Metabolism* 10 (2013): 71.

Post, R. E., A. G. Mainous III, D. E. King, and K. N. Simpson. "Dietary Fiber for the Treatment of Type 2 Diabetes Mellitus: A Meta-Analysis." *Journal of the American Board of Family Medicine* 25, no. 1 (February 2012): 16–23.

Rennard, B. O., R. F. Ertl, G. L. Gossman, R. A. Robbins, and S. I. Rennard. "Chicken Soup Inhibits Neutrophil Chemotaxis In Vitro." *CHEST* 118, no. 4 (October 2000): 1150–57.

Ricci, J. A., et al. "Fatigue in the U.S. Workforce: Prevalence and Implications for Lost Productive Work Time." *Journal of Occupational and Environmental Medicine* 49, no. 1 (January 2007): 1–10.

Rodriguez, N. R., N. M. DiMarco, and S. Langley. "Nutrition and Athletic Performance." *Medscape*, March 2009; http://www.medscape.com/viewarticle/717046.

Roman, M. J., and J. E. Salmon. "Cardiovascular Manifestations of Rheumatologic Diseases." *Circulation* 116 (2007): 2346–55.

Samocha-Bonet, D., et al. "Metabolically Healthy and Unhealthy Obese—The 2013 Stock Conference Report." *Obesity Reviews* 15, no. 9 (July 2014): 697–708; http://onlinelibrary.wiley.com/enhanced/doi/10.1111/obr.12199/.

Schmidt, K., et al. "Prebiotic Intake Reduces the Waking Cortisol Response and Alters Emotional Bias in Healthy Volunteers." *Psychopharmacology* 232, no. 10 (December 2014): 1793–801.

Schnoll, R., D. Burshteyn, and J. Cea-Aravena. "Nutrition in the Treatment of Attention-Deficit Hyperactivity Disorder: A Neglected but Important Aspect." *Applied Psychophysiology and Biofeedback* 28, no. 1 (March 2003): 63–75.

Scholz, A. "Cellulite Can't Simply Be Rubbed Away! Whey and Aminos as 'Make-up from the inside.'" *German Association for Sports Nutrition and Nutritional Supplements* 3 (2004).

Schwarz, S., C. Knorr, H. Geiger, and P. Flachenecker. "Complementary and Alternative Medicine for Multiple Sclerosis." *Multiple Sclerosis Journal* 14, no. 8 (September 2008): 1113–19.

Setiawan, E., et al. "Role of Translocator Protein Density, a Marker of Neuroinflammation, in the Brain During Major Depressive Episodes." *JAMA Psychiatry* 72, no. 3 (2015): 268–75.

Smith, S. M., and W. W. Vale. "The Role of Hypothalamic-Pituitary-Adrenal Axis in Neuroendocrine Responses to Stress." *Dialogues in Clinical Neuroscience* 8, no. 4 (2006): 383–95.

Suez, J., et al. "Artificial Sweeteners Induce Glucose Intolerance by Altering the Gut Microbiota." *Nature,* 514 (October 2014): 181–86.

Tillisch, K., et al. "Consumption of Fermented Milk Product with Probiotic Modulates Brain Activity." *Gastroenterology* 144, no. 7 (2013):1394–401.e4.

Trafton, A. "Inside the Adult ADHD Brain: Brain Scans Differentiate Adults Who Have Recovered from Childhood ADHD and Those Whose Difficulties Linger." McGovern Institute for brain research at MIT, website posting, June 2014; http://mcgovern.mit.edu/news/news/inside-the-adult-adhd-brain/.

Turnbaugh, P. J., et al. "The Effect of Diet on the Human Gut Microbiome: A Metagenomic Analysis in Humanized Gnotobiotic Mice." *Science Translational Medicine* 1, no. 6 (November 2009): 6–14.

Villegas, R., et al. "Vegetable But Not Fruit Consumption Reduces the Risk of Type 2 Diabetes in Chinese Women." *Journal of Nutrition* 138, no. 3 (March 2008): 574–80.

Vincent, G., et al. "Changes in Mitochondrial Function and Mitochondria Associated Protein Expression in Response to 2 Weeks of High Intensity Interval Training." *Front Physiology* 6 (February 24, 2015): 51.

Walker, A. F., R. W. Middleton, and O. Petrowicz. "Artichoke Leaf Extract Reduces Symptoms of Irritable Bowel Syndrome in a Post-marketing Surveillance Study." *Phytotherapy Research* 15, no. 1 (January 2011): 58–61; http://online library.wiley.com/doi/10.1002/1099-.

Williams, G., III. "Every Time You Wake Up, Your Body Must Restart Its Engine. Here Are Some Ways To Help Rev It Up." *American Health Magazine-Washington Post Writers Group*, November 1986: http://articles.chicagotribune .com/1986-11-19/entertainment/8603270048_1_wake-up-brain-cells.

Williams, C. "Is Depression a Kind of Allergic Reaction?" *The Guardian*, January 2015; http://www.theguardian.com/lifeandstyle/2015/jan/04/depression -allergic-reaction-inflammation-immune-system?CMP=share_btn_fb.

Williams, P. G. "The Benefits of Breakfast Cereal Consumption: A Systematic Review of the Evidence Base." *Advances in Nutrition* 5 (September 2014): 6365–735.

Wolever, T. M., D. J. Jenkins, L. U. Thompson, G. S. Wong, and R. G. Josse. "Effect of Canning on the Blood Glucose Response to Beans in Patients with Type 2 Diabetes." *Human Nutrition, Clinical Nutrition* 42, no. 2 (1987): 135–40.

Yancy, Jr., W. S., M. K. Olsen, J. R. Guyton, R. P. Bakst, and E. C. Westman. "A Low-Carbohydrate, Ketogenic Diet versus a Low-Fat Diet to Treat Obesity and Hyperlipidemia: A Randomized, Controlled Trial." *Annals of Internal Medicine* 140, no. 10 (May 2004): 769–77.

Zajac, A., et al. "The Effects of a Ketogenic Diet on Exercise Metabolism and Physical Performance in Off-Road Cyclists." *Nutrients* 6, no. 7 (2014): 2493–508.

Zheng, P., et al. "Identification and Validation of Urinary Metabolite Biomarkers for Major Depressive Disorder." *Molecular & Cellular Proteomics* 12, no. 1 (January 2013): 207–14.

Zukier, Z, J. A. Solomon, and M. J. Hamadeh. "The Role of Nutrition in Mental Health: Attention Deficit Hyperactivity Disorder (ADHD)." *Nutrition and ADHD*, 2010. http://www.mindingourbodies.ca/sites/default/files/adhd_and _nutrition_20100821.pdf.

Notes

CHAPTER 1

1 B.M. Burton-Freeman et al., "Whole Food versus Supplement: Comparing the Clinical Evidence of Tomato Intake and Lycopene Supplementation on Cardiovascular Risk Factors," *Advances in Nutrition* 5 (2014): 457–85.

2 National Institute of Diabetes and Digestive and Kidney Diseases, Division of Diabetes, Endocrinology, & Metabolic Diseases (DEM), http://www.niddk.nih.gov/about-niddk/offices-divisions/division-diabetes-endocrinology-metabolic-diseases/Pages/default.aspx.

3 National Heart, Lung, and Blood Institute, "What Is Metabolic Syndrome?" Online article, National Institutes of Health, http://www.nhlbi.nih.gov/health/health-topics/topics/ms.

4 S. W. Coppack et al., "Adipose Tissue Metabolism in Obesity: Lipase Action in vivo Before and After a Mixed Meal," *Metabolism: Clinical and Experimental* 41 no. 3 (1992): 264–72.

5 D. H. Pesta et al., "The Effects of Caffeine, Nicotine, Ethanol, and Tetrahydrocannabinol on Exercise Performance," *Nutrition & Metabolism* 10 (2013): 71.

6 A. Zajac et al., "The Effects of a Ketogenic Diet on Exercise Metabolism and Physical Performance in Off-Road Cyclists," *Nutrients* 6, no. 7 (2014): 2493–508.

CHAPTER 2

7 Linda Brookes, "Significant New Definitions, Publications, Risks, Benefits: American Heart Association and National Heart, Lung and Blood Institute Update ATP III Definition of Metabolic Syndrome," from *Hypertension Highlights*, a Medscape Cardiology article. http://www.medscape.org/viewarticle/514644.

8 B. S. McEwan, "Physiology and Neurobiology of Stress and Metabolic Adaptation: Central Role of the Brain," *Physiological Reviews* 87, no. 3 (2007): 873–904.

9 Endocrine Society, "Studies on Metabolic Adaptation," *Endocrinology* 21 (2013); http://press.endocrine.org/doi/abs/10.1210/endo-21-2-169.

10 A. Gonzalez et al., "The Mind-Body-Microbial Continuum," *Dialogues in Clinical Neuroscience* 13, no. 1 (2011): 55–62.

11 J. Alcock et al., "Is Eating Behavior Manipulated by the Gastrointestinal Microbiota? Evolutionary Pressures and Potential Mechanisms," *Bioessays* 36, no. 10 (October 2014): 940–49.

12 D. S. Goldstein, "Adrenal Responses to Stress," *Cellular and Molecular Neurobiology* 30, no. 8 (2010): 1433–40.

13 S. M. Smith and W. W. Vale, "The Role of Hypothalamic-Pituitary-Adrenal Axis in Neuroendocrine Responses to Stress," *Dialogues in Clinical Neuroscience* 8, no. 4 (2006): 383–95.

CHAPTER 5

14 Mark Hyman, "This Gut Condition Affects One in Six People—And Is Entirely Treatable," http://drhyman.com/blog/2015/04/09/this-gut-condition-affects-one-in-six-people-and-is-entirely-treatable/#close.

15 C. Canavan et al., "The Epidemiology of Irritable Bowel Syndrome," *Clinical Epidemiology* 6 (2014): 71–80.

16 See "The Most Common OTC Medications," at http://www.dailyrx.com/over-counter-medications-most-common-us-include-cough-cold-and-allergy-otc-remedies.

CHAPTER 9

17 E. Setiawan et al., "Role of Translocator Protein Density, a Marker of Neuroinflammation, in the Brain During Major Depressive Episodes," *JAMA Psychiatry* 72, no. 3 (2015): 268–75.

18 J. C. Felger and F. E. Lotrich, "Inflammatory Cytokines in Depression: Neurobiological Mechanisms and Therapeutic Implications," *Neuroscience* 246 (2013): 199–229.

19 K. Schmidt et al., "Prebiotic Intake Reduces the Waking Cortisol Response and Alters Emotional Bias in Healthy Volunteers," *Psychopharmacology*, posted 2014, http://link.springer.com/article/10.1007/s00213-014-3810-0/fulltext.html; also, K. Tillisch et al., "Consumption of Fermented Milk Product With Probiotic Modulates Brain Activity," *Gastroenterology* 144, no. 7 (2013): 1394–401.e4.

20 P. Zheng et al., "Identification and Validation of Urinary Metabolite Biomarkers for Major Depressive Disorder," *Molecular & Cellular Proteomics*, posted 2012, http://www.mcponline.org/content/early/2012/10/30/mcp.M112.021816.full.pdf+html.

21 G. E. Hodes et al., "Individual Differences in the Peripheral Immune System Promote Resilience versus Susceptibility to Social Stress," *CrossMark: Proceedings of the National Academy of Sciences of the United States of America* 111, no. 45: 16136–41.

CHAPTER 11

22 A. Kaya et al., "Autoantibodies in Heart Failure and Cardiac Dysfunction," *Circulation Research* 110 (2012): 145–58.
23 M. Abu-Shakra et al., "Cancer and Autoimmunity: Autoimmune and Rheumatic Features in Patients with Malignancies," *Annals of the Rheumatic Diseases* 60 (2001): 433–41.

Index

snacks (*cont'd*)
    for mood and cognition repair, 187,
      191
    per day, 66–67
soda, 254
Soups
    Hawaiian Chicken, 120
    Vegetarian Bean, 188–89
spices, 84
Spinach
    Green Smoothie, 140
    -Mushroom Wrap, 110–20
    Poached Egg Sandwich with
      Blueberries, 142–43
    and Steak Salad, 162
    Veggie Bagel, 233
SSRIs, 195
statin drugs, 154, 155, 167–68, 200
Stews
    Dumpling and Turkey, 186–88
    Grilled Chicken and Vegetable,
      143–44
    Slow Cooker Turkey Chili, 185
stimulant dependence, 108
stomach pains, 92
stool analysis test, 103
stools, 92
stool softeners, 90
stress
    chronic, 112–13
    hormones, 112–13, 130
    physiological responses to, 36–38
    -reduction methods, 124, 146,
      238–39
sugar, 56–57, 200, 201, 254
sugar cravings, 108, 173, 201, 203
suicidal thoughts, 173
sweat resistance, 153

talk therapy, 191
testes, 135
testosterone, 125–26, 131, 134, 147,
    153
thirst, 203
thyroid, 109, 135, 147, 193–94, 220

Tomatoes
    Chicken Marinara Pasta, 214
    Grilled Chicken and Vegetable Stew,
      143–44
    Haylie's Fermented Salsa, 190–91
    lycopene in, 11–12
    Slow Cooker Turkey Chili, 185
toxins, 194, 225, 254
tremors, 173
triglycerides, 24, 76, 151, 153, 203
Turkey
    Chili, Slow Cooker, 185
    Cucumber Submarine Sandwich,
      236
    and Dumpling Stew, 186–88

ulcers, 93, 103
urinalysis, 218
urination, 204
urine leakage, 130

vaginal dryness, 130
vegetables
    cultured or fermented, 182
    on Foundation Food List, 81
    frozen, 254
    Quick Pickled Veggies, 189–90
    raw, 160
    serving size, 81
viral infections, 92, 225
vitamin D
    lab tests for, 147, 167
    low, health issues from, 109, 133–35,
      153, 204

water intake, 68
water retention, 153
weepiness, 130
weight gain
    from carbs, 108, 204
    from hormone imbalance, 130
    losing, setting goal for, 19
    midsection, 203

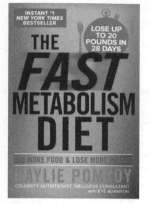
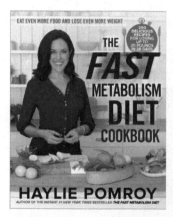
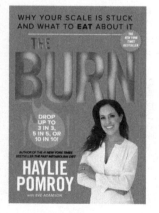
 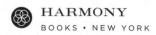

✕ HAYLIE POMROY
Real food, real people, real change.

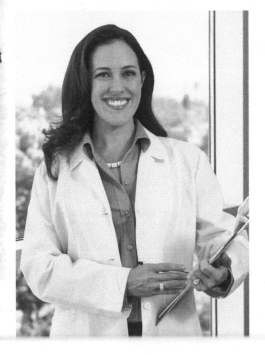

Come be my guest and explore our life-changing website!

Welcome! I'm so excited to have you be my guest on this exclusive site where you can get the tools and answers you need. You're making the best decision to empower yourself.

Membership guarantees you more than just access to my site or a few e-mails. Membership is a promise from me to you that you're a top priority and a valued member of the community. The benefits are immense!

Here's what you'll receive when becoming a member:

- Support and encouragement from others who share your same struggles
- Rapid answers to your questions and concerns
- Practical and tangible solutions and tools to address the problems you are facing
- 10% off store purchases at hayliepomroy.com to supplement your health

---

GET YOUR FREE 7-DAY MEMBERSHIP TRIAL TODAY!
Use coupon code: BEMYGUEST
Offer expires February 23, 2017

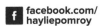 facebook.com/ hayliepomroy   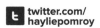 twitter.com/ hayliepomroy   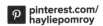 pinterest.com/ hayliepomroy   youtube: hayliepomroy   instagram: hayliepomroy

www.HayliePomroy.com